Age-Defying
Fitness

Information contained within this book is not to be construed as medical guidance. Before beginning any exercise program, please consult your physician or physical therapist.

Published by
Peachtree Publishers
1700 Chattahoochee Avenue
Atlanta, Georgia 30318-2112

www.peachtree-online.com

Book and cover design by Regina Dalton-Fischel and Loraine Joyner
Composition by Robin Sherman and Melanie McMahon Ives
Production editor: Kathy Landwehr

Printed in the United States of America
10 9 8 7 6 5 4

Library of Congress Cataloging-in-Publication Data

Moffat, Marilyn.
  Age-defying fitness : making the most of your body for the rest of your life /
by Marilyn Moffat and Carole B. Lewis.— 1st ed.
     p. cm.
  ISBN 978-1-56145-389-4 book only
  ISBN 978-1-56145-333-7 book and Thera-band®
1. Exercise. 2. Physical fitness. 3. Aging—Physiological aspects. 4. Longevity.
I. Title: Age defying fitness. II. Lewis, Carole Bernstein. III. Title.
RA781.M64 2005
613.7'1—dc22
                                    2005026704

Age-Defying Fitness

Making the Most of Your Body for the Rest of Your Life

■■■■■■

Marilyn Moffat, PT, DPT, PhD, FAPTA

Carole B. Lewis, PT, DPT, PhD, FAPTA

with contributions from Jean Marie McAndrew

Photographs by Linda Schaefer

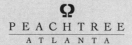

PEACHTREE
ATLANTA

To my family who have always reminded me of what is important in life; to my colleagues, students, patients, and clients who have taught me so much and made me realize what insight and passion mean in realizing one's goals; and to my early school and college mentors who instilled in me a love of exercise and physical activity. —*M. M.*

Ties with family, friends, and colleagues are the fabric of my life. The inspirations that you have provided me are the fuel that keeps me going. I would like to dedicate this book to each of you. Your input, support, and love have inspired me to undertake what is a very important work, in my eyes. I have always wanted to write on the subject of aging and fitness, and thanks to each of you my dream has come true.

Thank you for being a part of the process. The tapestry that is our interwoven lives is reflected in the pages of this book—a permanent record of the bond that holds each of you in a place in my heart. —*C. L.*

Contents

Chapter 1: Assessing Your Body

Chapter 2: Posture

Chapter 3: Strength

Chapter 4: Balance

Chapter 5: Flexibility

Chapter 6: Endurance

Chapter 7: Putting It All Together

A NOTE FROM THE AUTHORS

As physical therapists, we look at the body as if it were a truly remarkable machine, which it is. To keep this machine in proper working order—tuned-up, so to speak—and to age gracefully and be physically happy, it's important for you to address what we call the 5 domains of fitness—posture, strength, balance, flexibility, and endurance.

We wrote this book because we agreed that it was time for us to share our clinical experience and research expertise about the benefits of exercise. We encourage you to read the first chapter carefully because it sets the stage for the rest of the book, explaining why changes are occurring in your body in each of the 5 domains and how they are affected by activity. General, simple tests in this first chapter help you assess your capabilities in the 5 domains. The chapters that follow guide you in exploring and assessing your current level of physical fitness in each domain. Based on the results of your assessments, you can then devise a personalized exercise plan to help you achieve and maintain your maximum potential.

We hope our book will inspire and motivate you to do something good and long lasting for yourself: exercise. The step-by-step photographs will make the challenge less daunting and the task more manageable. With AGE-DEFYING FITNESS, you have the tools you need to keep yourself fit and healthy. We wish you well.

Marilyn Moffat, PT, DPT, PhD, FAPTA, CSCS
Carole B. Lewis, PT, DPT, PhD, MPA, MSG, FAPTA, GCS

PHYSICAL THERAPY: FREQUENTLY ASKED QUESTIONS

What is a physical therapist?

A physical therapist is a professional practitioner whose examinations, interventions, and treatments are aimed at restoring, maintaining, and promoting optimal physical function. Physical therapists:

- Diagnose and manage movement disorders.

- Help people enhance their physical and functional abilities.

- Promote optimal wellness, fitness, and quality of life as it relates to movement and health.

- Help people prevent the onset, symptoms, and progression of impairments, functional limitations, and disabilities.

What special skills do physical therapists have?

Physical therapists are experts in exercise. They have in-depth knowledge about all forms of exercise—strengthening (isometrics, isokinetics, eccentric, concentric, progressive resistive), neuromuscular reeducation, stretching, relaxation, core stabilization, breathing, and aerobics—as they relate to movement, function, health, wellness, and fitness. They have undergone many hours of training in manual skills such as joint mobilization, massage, soft tissue work, and passive range of motion. They provide in-depth examination and interventions for faulty posture, body mechanics, and ergonomics. Their specialty is functional assessment and functional training. They are unmatched in assessing joint motion and testing the strength of individual muscles.

Where do physical therapists practice?

Physical therapists provide services in hospitals, outpatient clinics and offices, fitness centers, sports training facilities, rehabilitation facilities, retirement communities, nursing homes, transitional care units, extended care facilities, and hospices. They practice in school settings and playgrounds with children who have disabilities.

Many physical therapists make house calls, providing rehabilitation or exercise interventions to people in their homes. Physical therapists may practice in corporate or industrial health settings or other occupational environments. Some physical therapists teach in colleges and universities or conduct research.

What is the educational background of a physical therapist?

In the United States, physical therapists hold doctorates (DPT, or Doctor of Physical Therapy). Students first complete 4 years of undergraduate or baccalaureate education with a heavy science concentration (biology, chemistry, physics, and physiology) and then they enter a 3-year physical therapy program.

The physical therapist curriculum consists of study in the basic sciences, applied sciences, and clinical sciences. Students learn procedural interventions, the examination process, critical inquiry, and clinical decision making. Each program features about 1 full year of clinical practice in multiple settings.

Are there specialty areas in physical therapy?

Yes. They include orthopedics, neurology, sports physical therapy, geriatrics, pediatrics, clinical electrophysiology, and women's health. The American Physical Therapy Association offers specialty certification in several of these areas.

Are physical therapists licensed?

Physical therapists must be licensed to practice in the United States. To be licensed, therapists must graduate from a physical therapy curriculum that is accredited by the Commission on Accreditation of Physical Therapy Education and pass the national licensing exam in the state where they wish to practice.

Is there a national association for physical therapists?

The American Physical Therapy Association is the national organization representing physical therapists across the United States.

How can I locate a physical therapist?

The American Physical Therapy Association (www.apta.org) and many state physical therapy organizations maintain a list of physical therapists by geographical area. They are also listed in the yellow pages of your local telephone directory. Call one up and make an appointment.

Do I need a referral from a physician to consult a physical therapist?

You may seek an examination by a physical therapist in all but two states in the United States (Indiana and Alabama). In some states you may need a referral for treatment.

Are physical therapy services covered by insurance?

Most insurance plans cover physical therapy; however, as every plan is different, it's important to learn what your plan covers. Physical therapy coverage was written into the first Medicare legislation so it has been covered by that plan for many years. Medicaid also covers physical therapy services.

WHAT IS A THERA-BAND®?

Some of the exercises in this book call for the use of an elastic band called a Thera-band®. Thera-bands are used by physical therapists for conditioning, rehabilitation, and strength building. Used properly, Thera-bands provide both positive and negative force on your muscles, improving strength, range of motion, and cooperation of muscle groups.

You can use a Thera-band for some of the assessments and exercises in this book. Directions for its use are included where appropriate. You can even take it with you when you travel so you can maintain your training program wherever you are.

An offer for a free Thera-band is included in this book. (The postcard for ordering the band is bound into the book following the last page.) You can also purchase Thera-bands from many sources online and in retail stores. We will keep a list of suppliers on our website for your convenience: *www.agedefyingfitness.com.*

Thera-bands are available in 8 color-coded levels of resistance. The green band, which gives moderate resistance, is recommended for use with this book and is the one provided in the free offer. After some experience, you may wish to try another level of resistance. There are 3 bands offering less resistance and 4 offering greater. For more information about Thera-bands, visit *http://www.thera-band.com/resistive.html.*

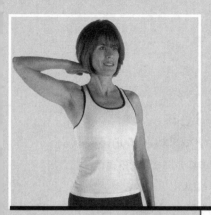

Chapter 1

■ ■ ■ ■ ■

Assessing Your Body

WHAT'S IN THIS CHAPTER?

■ ■ ■ ■ ■

SHOULD YOU CONSULT A PHYSICAL THERAPIST?

We strongly believe that if you are 50 or older, you should consult a physical therapist to help you get started with an exercise program. Physical therapists have specialized knowledge that will help you develop an effective and safe plan to use throughout your life. Your consultation may include the following:

- A review of your complete health and exercise-related history (This may be obtained in writing in advance or at the beginning of the visit.)
- An examination to screen your overall joint range of motion, muscle strength, body symmetry, weight, height, walking pattern, balance, coordination, blood pressure, heart rate, and respiratory rate.
- An assessment of your functional abilities at home, at work, and during leisure activities.

If need be, the therapist may perform more in-depth measures of your physical performance abilities. Grid photographs or a plumb line help measure posture limitations. A dynamometer accurately evaluates strength limitations, and a goniometer assesses flexibility or range-of-motion limitations. To measure balance limitations, a therapist may use the Berg Balance Scale or similar scales. An aerobic capacity test evaluates endurance limitations.

After a thorough examination, the physical therapist will map out a specific program for you. Another visit may be scheduled to assess your progress, answer your questions, and modify your plan as needed. As physical therapists, our goals are to help you become as independent as possible in your long-term fitness program and to assure that your program becomes a potent and positive factor in your life.

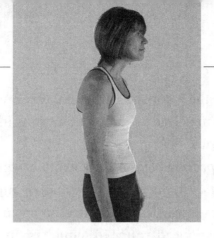

A QUICK QUIZ

□ Do you feel like you're not standing as straight and tall
 as you once did?
□ Is walking up a flight of stairs a strain at times?
□ Are you getting up from your chair more slowly
 than you used to?
□ Is it getting more difficult for you to look to the left and
 right while backing up your car?
□ Do you get stiff sitting through a long movie?
□ Is standing on 1 leg to put on your shoe difficult
 or impossible?
□ Do you trip or lose your balance more easily?
□ Does walking or jogging a distance take longer
 than it used to?

If you answered yes to any of these questions, read on.

AGE-RELATED PHYSICAL CHANGES

The human body is truly amazing. Mechanisms put in place as soon as
life begins help us grow and acquire various physical skills. Once the body
systems have fully matured, the changes brought about by aging com-
mence—in some systems, these changes begin as early as the teens.

Our physical well-being can be observed and measured through what
we call the 5 domains of fitness: posture, strength, balance, flexibility, and

endurance. Age affects the 5 domains in several ways. As you age, changes that are subtle at first may lead to major alterations in your physical performance capabilities.

The nice, tall, erect *posture* of youth all too often begins to change as early as the teen years. Prolonged sitting, using a computer, and carrying a heavy purse or briefcase may lead to changes in postural alignment, including a more forward head, rounded shoulders, an increase or decrease of the spinal curve in the lower back, and increased bending in the hips and knees. Poor posture can be exacerbated by a weakening or tightening in some of the neck and trunk muscles.

Strength declines with age. This decline is thought to be due to a combination of decreases in muscle fiber size and amount, nerve supply to the muscle, and overall energy supply and circulation.

Balance is also affected as you age. The tightening and weakening of muscles and decreased range of movement of joints can alter the body's ability to respond to a balance challenge. Decreased circulation can affect the brain's ability to help you stay balanced. A loss of nerve input causes a slowing in the body's ability to respond to balance situations. These changes make you increasingly prone to falls.

Loss of *flexibility* results from changes in the body's collagen structures. Collagen is a fibrous connective tissue that makes up about 30 percent of the protein in all of your body tissues (skin, muscle sheath, bone, tendons, ligament, cartilage). As you age, collagen fibers begin to stick together, causing connective tissue to become less elastic.

Age also affects *endurance,* the ability to perform an activity like walking or running for a prolonged period of time. Because you are less flexible and have weakened muscles, it takes more energy to remain physically active. Thus, your body tires more quickly than it did when you were younger. A loss of elasticity in the lungs and a slight stiffening of the air passageways can make breathing harder during endurance exercise.

Changes in blood vessel elasticity and a decrease in the maximum heart rate may also lead to potential losses in endurance.

The Amazing Antidote

The antidote to aging is activity. No matter what your age is now, no matter how inactive you have been, it is possible to increase your fitness and improve your posture, strength, balance, flexibility, and endurance. Inactivity magnifies age-related changes, but action maintains and increases your abilities in all 5 domains. Our plan of self-evaluation and exercises focused on your particular needs may show results within just a few weeks. We've seen it happen over and over in the lives of our clients and patients. It's not magic, but it is amazing.

As people get older, many of them slide into one of two categories, "weekend warriors" or "weekend worriers." "Warriors," who were usually athletic in their earlier years, participate in fairly intense sports on weekends after spending all week at a desk. These folks are prone to injuries. "Worriers" work nonstop and almost never exercise. If and when they do take a break, they may notice their bodies are stiff and slumping, and they feel listless.

You might be a "warrior" or a "worrier," or you might be like Wendy or James.

Meet Wendy

Wendy is a 48-year-old woman with a high-powered career in Washington, DC, and she is single-handedly raising 2 teenagers. Wendy's weekends are rarely times of rest and relaxation; housework, errands, time with her children, and—often—weekend work projects fill her days "off." Wendy notices her posture sagging as well as feelings of exhaustion, stiffness, and unsteadiness. She also notices that it's a little difficult to turn her head while she backs her car out of a parking space. Wendy makes an appointment with her doctor who suggests muscle relaxants and exercise.

Wendy resolves to join an exercise group. She begins with a step class enthusiastically recommended by a friend and finds she has more energy, but she feels stiff and is sore on the days after class. She abandons the step class due to her stiffness and signs up for a yoga class, but she doesn't enjoy that either. She can't keep up with the more experienced people in the class, and she feels like she's not as strong or as flexible as she needs to be. She drops out.

You may be like Wendy. She has small declines in all 5 areas of physical health. A few daily exercises and helpful tips might make her feel and look better. But she needs the *right* regimen.

Meet James

James is a 65-year-old, semiretired editor. In his youth he played a variety of sports from football to tennis, and he continued to play tennis weekly into his fifties until a series of injuries made him hang up his racquet. Now he fills his days with working part-time, watching television, and reading the newspaper. His editing work is sedentary.

Lately, he hasn't had as much energy as usual. He feels stiff when he wakes up in the morning, loses his balance at times, gets winded when climbing stairs, and walks more slowly than he used to. In addition, he's had a little difficulty maintaining his balance when dressing, bending over to tie his shoes, and bending his arm around to wash the middle of his back. James gets his heart rate and blood pressure checked regularly, and his doctor told him he is healthy but could use some exercise.

James doesn't know much about exercise, especially about what type of exercise would be most beneficial for him. Plus, he doesn't want to join a gym because he feels foolish exercising in front of others.

James may be like you. He is experiencing some physical problems, and he needs some good information and suggestions on what he can do to help himself.

Wendy and James are people who have made a commitment to exercise. You'll hear more about them in chapters 2 through 7, and you'll see how they used the exercises in this book to improve their fitness.

GETTING STARTED

What will make you—personally—start and continue your own program toward healthy physical performance? We hope learning as much as you can about exercise motivation and determination will help you become a dedicated exerciser.

Behavior is governed by expectations and incentives. The likelihood that you will adopt the healthy behavior of life-long exercise depends primarily upon these 3 conditions:

- You perceive your health is threatened.
- You expect your exercise program will make you healthier or feel significantly better.
- You expect you can change your previous lifestyle and incorporate exercise into your life.

HOW TO USE THIS BOOK

Have you ever attempted a new fitness program without assessing your current capabilities? If so, you probably had no way of knowing where you were when you started. The first step to becoming a new and improved you is to assess your physical performance. As physical therapists, we know the importance of establishing baseline measurements. Objective measures of the 5 domains provided in each chapter will show you where you need to target your efforts. The tests give you immediate, specific, and usable information for determining your current level of physical function, and the recorded results will enable you to measure your improvement. Once you have identified your specific areas for concentration, we'll give you the tools to develop your individualized program—specific exercises that target problem areas.

At the end of the assessment section in each chapter, you'll find a blank exercise prescription. Make a photocopy, fill in the exercises specifically recommended for you, and use it as a bookmark to keep your place as you do the exercises in the chapter. Complete a new assessment in 2 months and compare your results. These plans will help mark your progress over time.

We suggest that you return to this chapter and retest yourself every 2 months as a general measure of your improvement. You may also retest yourself more thoroughly in each of the 5 specific domain chapters.

ASSESSING THE FIVE DOMAINS

TEST 1: POSTURE

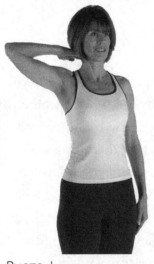

PHOTO 1

1. Stand with your head and back against a wall and your feet 10 to 12 inches away from the wall.

2. While maintaining this position, straighten your back so that your neck is as close to the wall as possible. Be sure to keep your entire back and buttocks against the wall throughout the test.

3. Place one hand behind your neck with your palm flat and facing down. See how many fingers you can fit between the curve in your neck and the wall (photo 1).

RESULT (Check the one that applies to you)

a.___My head does not touch the wall.

b.___My head touches the wall and I can fit 5 fingers behind my neck.

c.___My head touches the wall and I can fit 4 fingers behind my neck.

d.___My head touches the wall and I can fit 3 fingers behind my neck.

e.___My head touches the wall and I can fit 2 fingers behind my neck.

f.___ My head touches the wall and I can fit 1 finger behind my neck.

g.___There is no space between my neck and the wall.

If statement a, b, c, or d applies to you, read chapter 2 on Posture. If your neck is more than two fingers away from the wall, you hold your head too far forward or you round your upper back. Your posture is not in appropriate alignment, and you should complete the full posture assessment in chapter 2.

Posture difficulties are truly a sign of the times. Most people spend time every day at the computer or in front of the television; no wonder their posture suffers. However, poor posture is not irreversible. The body is very pliable at any age, and the program for improving posture is easy to do.

If you answered yes to statements e, f, or g, you still may benefit from the material in chapter 2.

We tell our clients and patients to notice television and film stars; many of them exhibit perfect posture, especially if they are playing heroes or heroines. The small amount of effort required and the tips you will find in the posture chapter merit the time it will take to read it. A little information and effort can make a huge difference in your posture and how you look and feel.

TEST 2: STRENGTH

This test is a well-researched method of measuring lower body strength and the values are age and gender based (see Chart 1 on page 11). You will need a sturdy chair and a stopwatch or clock with a second hand.

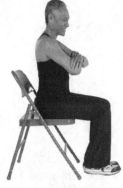

1. Sit barefoot or in sneakers or other flat shoes in a good supporting armless chair. Do not lean back.

2. Place your arms across your chest. Do not use them for help throughout the test (photo 1).

3. Start the clock and time how long it takes you to rise to a complete standing position (photo 2) and sit back down 10 times in a row. Do this as quickly as you can.

PHOTO 1

4. Stop the clock.

RESULT

Time required to complete 10 full stands:_____

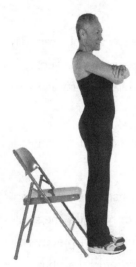

Find your age and gender in Chart 1 to see how much time it should take you to complete the test. If you are slower than average for your age, read chapter 3 on Strength. If you are average or faster for your age, take the other tests in chapter 3 to ensure that you maintain (and perhaps increase) your strength.

PHOTO 2

Chart I

AVERAGE PREDICTED TIME FOR 10 FULL STANDS
FOR EACH AGE AND GENDER GROUP

Age In years	Women Average in seconds	Men Average in seconds
30	12.6	10.8
35	13.4	11.7
40	14.3	12.7
45	15.1	13.7
50	15.9	14.7
55	16.8	15.6
60	17.6	16.6
65	18.4	17.6
70	19.3	18.5
75	20.1	19.5
80	20.9	20.5
85	21.8	21.5

Efforts to improve your strength will pay off. When you feel strong, you also feel more confident. Many studies have shown that reduction in strength in older adults is often the result of decreased activity. Muscle strength is often lost through disuse and can be regained. Most of our clients and patients report they notice a difference in strength within 2 weeks of beginning a program; they find activities like walking, lifting, and getting out of chairs are noticeably easier.

We can't help but notice that our older clients and patients who maintain a high level of physical activity are stronger than many of those who are younger and less active.

TEST 3: BALANCE

To do this test you will either need to hold a stopwatch or have another person time you. **Caution:** Be sure there is a counter or piece of furniture near enough to reach to steady yourself if necessary, or ask a friend to spot you to ensure your safety while performing this test.

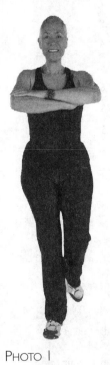

1. Stand up straight, wearing sneakers or other flat shoes. Place your arms across your chest. Raise 1 leg off the floor, start the stopwatch, and close your eyes (photo 1).

2. Remain standing on 1 leg. Stop the watch if you uncross your arms, tilt your trunk to either side more than 45 degrees, move your stationary leg, or touch your raised leg to the floor.

3. Repeat the test standing on the other leg.

RESULT

Time able to stand on right leg with eyes closed: _____

Time able to stand on left leg with eyes closed: _____

Photo 1

If you cannot stand with your eyes closed at least 5 seconds on each side, read chapter 5 on Balance. If you are able to stand for 5 seconds or more, take the additional tests in chapter 5 to check for other possible balance problems.

Balance is an area of physical fitness that is often overlooked. When our clients and patients work on this area, they get fast, effective results. One of us developed a program for a woman who loved to travel, was increasingly afraid of falling, and had very limited time to exercise. She was given 2 exercises to be done 3 times a week for 8 weeks. After 2 months, she received a perfect balance score.

Perhaps you have great balance on 1 leg, but find walking on uneven surfaces or bending over to be difficult. In chapter 5 we provide exercises to target the very specific areas you need to ensure you don't focus your energies or activities on exercises that are only marginally helpful. After practicing these exercises, our clients and patients who have needed canes or other balance aids are astonished at how quickly they can function without them.

TEST 4: FLEXIBILITY

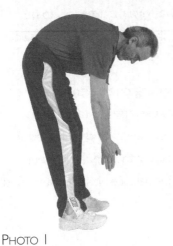

1. Stand with your knees straight and your arms hanging by your side.

2. Bend forward from the waist (photo 1). Do your middle fingers touch the floor?

RESULT

_____YES, my middle fingers touch the floor.

_____NO, my middle fingers are more than 2 inches from the floor.

PHOTO 1

If your middle fingers do not touch the floor, read chapter 4 on Flexibility. Even if your fingertips do touch the floor, take the additional flexibility tests found in chapter 4. You may not notice how tight your muscles are, since strength and endurance issues may affect your function more overtly. However, being less than optimally flexible can make you walk or move in ways that are neither safe nor comfortable.

While older muscle may lose some of its elasticity, it often just needs to be stretched. Even occasional gentle stretching is well worth the effort. Stretching appropriately will yield results within several weeks. Even after 1 or 2 sessions, some patients report that stretching feels good and helps them to relax.

TEST 5: ENDURANCE

A simple walk or run is the best test for establishing your endurance capability, which is really an assessment of your cardiovascular and pulmonary fitness. You can go to a track or other place where the miles are marked, or measure the distance using a pedometer or your car's odometer. **Caution:** If you have not been exercising regularly, test yourself with the walk test; do not run.

Timed Walk/Run Test

This test was validated for a fit population. If you have not been regularly performing endurance exercise, you may find that your results fall into the poor to fair range. Don't be disheartened. You can improve your endurance with conditioning. If you prefer, you may use the Rockport Walking Test on page 241 instead. Before taking that test, you must measure your resting heart rate and final heart rate.

1. Set the stopwatch for 12 minutes and begin walking/running on the measured route. **Caution:** Pay attention to how you feel. If the exercise begins to feel hard or stressful, turn off the stopwatch, slow down, and continue to walk while you cool down. You may want to try this test again in 2 days. If you still feel that it is too stressful, make an appointment to see your doctor.

2. When the time is up, record your distance. Assess your results, using the averages in Chart 2 on page 16.

Distance Run Test

1. Run 1.5 miles on the measured route. **Caution:** Pay attention to how you feel. If the exercise begins to feel hard or stressful, stop running, slow down, and walk while you cool down. In 2 days, try the Timed Walk/Run test.

2. Record the time it took you to run 1.5 miles. Assess your results, using the running averages in Chart 3 on page 17.

Chart 2

WALKING/RUNNING DISTANCE AVERAGES
FOR THE 12-MINUTE TIMED WALK/RUN TEST

For each age group, the range of expected miles in 12 minutes is given for both females (F) and males (M)

Fitness Category	Gender	30–39 yrs	40–49 yrs	50–59 yrs	60+ yrs
I. Very Poor	F	< 0.94	< 0.88	< 0.84	< 0.78
	M	< 1.18	< 1.14	< 1.03	< 0.87
II. Poor	F	0.95–1.05	0.88–0.98	0.84–0.93	0.78–0.86
	M	1.18–1.30	1.14–1.24	1.03–1.16	0.87–1.02
III. Fair	F	1.06–1.18	0.99–1.11	0.94–1.05	0.87–0.98
	M	1.31–1.45	1.25–1.39	1.17–1.30	1.03–1.20
IV. Good	F	1.19–1.29	1.12–1.24	1.06–1.18	0.99–1.09
	M	1.46–1.56	1.40–1.53	1.31–1.44	1.21–1.32
V. Excellent	F	1.30–1.39	1.25–1.34	1.19–1.30	1.10–1.18
	M	1.57–1.69	1.54–1.65	1.45–1.58	1.33–1.55
VI. Superior	F	> 1.40	> 1.35	> 1.31	> 1.19
	M	> 1.70	> 1.66	> 1.59	> 1.56

> means greater than and < means less than

Use a flat surface (e.g., oval track, shopping mall). Do not eat a heavy meal or smoke for 2–3 hours prior to the test. Warm up with a very easy walk/run first. To attain a realistic estimate of your fitness level, walk/run as quickly as seems reasonable for you during the 12-minute test. Cool down with a very easy walk of about 5 minutes to prevent pooling of the blood in the legs. The best results are achieved by doing a practice walk/run first so you know how to pace yourself.

Chart 3

RUNNING TIME AVERAGES FOR 1.5-MILE DISTANCE RUN

Males

	Age 30–39	Age 40–49	Age 50–59	Age 60-69	Age 70–79
Superior	≤ 8:07	≤ 8:35	≤ 9:45	≤11:00	≤12:20
Excellent	8:08–10:01	8:36–10:47	9:46–12:01	11:01–13:22	12:21–14:37
Good	10:02–11:39	10:48–12:20	12:02–13:47	13:23–14:59	14:38–16:27
Fair	11:40–12:51	12:21–13:46	13:48–14:54	15:00–16:16	16:28–17:29
Poor	12:52–14:23	13:47–15:07	14:55–16:22	16:17–17:41	17:30–19:02
Very Poor	14:24+	15:08+	16:23+	17:42+	19:03+

Females

	Age 30–39	Age 40–49	Age 50–59	Age 60-69	Age 70–79
Superior	≤10:44	≤11:20	≤13:13	≤14:21	≤14:24
Excellent	10:45–12:50	11:21–13:35	13:14–14:54	14:22–15:56	14:25–16:43
Good	12:51–14:23	13:36–14:57	14:55–16:15	15:57–17:06	16:44–18:00
Fair	14:24–15:25	14:58–16:22	16:16–17:14	17:07–18:00	18:01–18:59
Poor	15:26–16:48	16:23–17:29	17:15–18:23	18:01–19:02	19:00–19:56
Very Poor	16:49+	17:30+	18:24+	19:03+	19:57+

≤ means less than or equal to

Use a measured distance of 1.5 miles on a flat surface (e.g., oval track). Do not eat a heavy meal or smoke for 2–3 hours prior to the test. Warm up (walking, jogging) first. Cover the distance as rapidly as possible to attain a realistic estimate of your fitness level. If you cannot run the entire distance, walk until you can continue running again. Record time in minutes and seconds. Cool down by walking about 5 minutes to prevent blood pooling in your legs. The best results are achieved by doing a practice run first so you know how to pace yourself.

RESULTS

For Timed Walkers/Runners

■ Distance covered in 12 minutes: _____.

Use Chart 2 to compare your distance with the established norms for your gender and age.

■ If you could not walk for 12 minutes, record your time and the distance covered. If you use the Rockport Walking Test on page 241, record your Resting and Final Heart Rates.

Time: _____ Distance: _____ RHR: _____ FHR: _____

For Distance Runners

■ Time to run 1.5 miles: _____.

Use Chart 3 to compare your time with the established norms for your gender and age.

■ If you could not complete the 1.5-mile run using the time parameters in Chart 3, go back and retest yourself using the 12-minute walking/running test. (See Chart 2.)

Time: _____ Distance: _____

If your results are below the norms, the information in chapter 6 could work miracles in your life. Endurance is important. It gives you the vim and vigor to get through the day. You may blame stress and psychological concerns for your lack of energy, but if you exercise and keep your endurance at or above the norms for your gender and age, you'll find you feel much better. Chapter 6 offers additional tests that evaluate cardiovascular and pulmonary fitness and suggests a variety of ways to keep endurance exercises fresh and interesting.

We have helped thousands of women and men of all ages embark on the road to fitness. We can help you too.

The older you get, the more difficult it is to change, but it's not impossible. We have tried to make the exercises in this book straightforward, easy to understand, and simple to do at any age. We believe that you can master these exercises and feel confident about your exercise abilities. Don't be afraid to try.

When you feel better about yourself, you're more likely to exercise. The good news is that if you can grin and bear it at first, exercise is proven to help improve your mood and self-esteem. We provide a variety of exercises so you can begin with the ones you like best and modify them as you progress; however, we do give you suggestions on how to get started.

6 TIPS FOR SUCCESS

Starting an exercise program can be difficult, but you can do it! Use these 6 tips to help you succeed:

- **Be confident.** We believe in you, so you should believe in yourself.
- **Think of past successes.** Focus on them if you feel an urge to stop.
- **Start slowly.** That way you will not incur any unnecessary muscle soreness and you will begin to feel better about your abilities.
- **Proceed carefully.** Don't take things to the next level until you have successfully mastered your first program.
- **Monitor your performance.** Think of others who have failed and notice how you are different from them. Think of others who have succeeded and concentrate on your similarities to them.

■ **Enlist the support of family or friends.** They will help you keep going and make your exercise program both social and healthy. Try to get a friend or family member to exercise with you.

WHAT'S STOPPING YOU?

It is also important to recognize the forces that may be stopping you from exercising. The most basic reason for not doing something is fear. Here are 4 common fears that might prevent you from exercising, and ways to help you conquer those fears:

■ **Fear of rejection.** These exercises are for you and no one else. Rejection should not be an issue.

■ **Fear of embarrassment or looking foolish.** If you are concerned about what others will think, begin exercising by yourself. Once you start looking and feeling better, you will be less worried about other people watching you.

■ **Fear of wasted effort.** All health-related research is clear: exercise has significant benefits.

■ **Fear of failure or poor performance.** This book is for you, and you will be your own judge. Be gentle with yourself; very few people perform like experts when they begin an exercise program. Even if you occasionally feel discouraged, it's important never to give up.

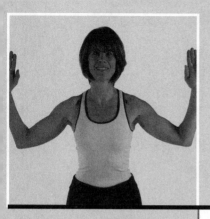

Chapter 2

Posture

WHAT'S IN THIS CHAPTER?

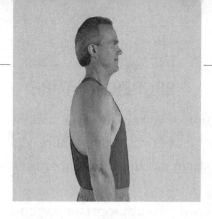

Stand up straight.
Admire the world.

—John Cheever

Your backbone is the key to good posture, and strong, solid posture is the backbone of feeling good and staying active. Many people, however, don't stand straight. Their heads droop, their shoulders round, their backs slump.

After work and on weekends, Richard, 51, could often be found reading or watching television on the big sofa in the den. He called it "relaxing." Working hard all day made him tired; he thought taking a well-deserved rest would make him feel better. But actually poor posture was wearing Richard out and contributing to his lack of energy. If anything, he was more tired on Monday morning than he had been on Friday night.

Over time, poor posture causes muscle weakness or tightness. Slumping while watching TV or using a computer may throw your spine out of alignment. Carrying heavy bags or uneven loads worsens the problem. Our parents and grandparents were onto something when they told us to sit up straight and stand erect. Perfecting your posture requires a lot of attention initially, but with practice it becomes second nature. Good habits build good posture, and good posture gives you more energy and fewer aches and pains.

PROPER POSTURE

Posture is the position of your body while standing, sitting, and performing daily tasks. When your body is properly aligned, it is well-balanced, with minimum stress and strain on supporting structures such as bones, ligaments, and muscles.

Good posture also provides appropriate positioning for your inner organs. Keeping your body straight gives your lungs the space they need for full expansion, and keeping your abdominal muscles tight provides support for intestinal and pelvic organs. Posture affects breathing and arm and neck movements. It even affects how your jaw works and the way you chew. To see just how important posture is to well-being, try these 3 simple movements.

- While standing, move your head forward; jut your chin out and increase the curve in the back of your neck. Round your shoulders and slump (photo 1). Now do each of these 4 movements:
  1. Take 3 deep breaths.
  2. Turn your head side-to-side.
  3. Raise both arms over your head.
  4. Tap your teeth together.

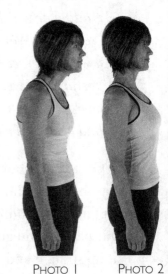

- Now pull your chin in, lengthen your neck, and look straight ahead. Bring your shoulders back and slightly down. Straighten your back, suck in your stomach (photo 2), and repeat the 4 movements.
  1. Take 3 deep breaths.
  2. Turn your head side-to-side.
  3. Raise both arms over your head.
  4. Tap your teeth together.

PHOTO 1   PHOTO 2

- Notice the difference. Do you feel how much easier it is to breathe deeply and move your head, arms, and jaw when you are well aligned?

Symmetry is an important aspect of good posture. Your body should be aligned equally side-to-side and back-to-front. When your body is in balance, it requires less work to stay erect. If your body is asymmetrical, some areas have to work more than others in order for you to maintain an upright position. Habitual, prolonged, unequal alignment results in more wear and tear on your body as you age.

POSTURE CHANGES

Posture does change over time, but many limitations that people associate with aging are actually due to inactivity. You may see older people with an almost goose-necked stance, head forward and shoulders severely rounded. But many younger people, especially those who spend a lot of time at their desks peering at computer monitors, exhibit these same postures earlier in life.

When Denise first visited her 80-year-old grandmother in the new nursing home, it didn't surprise her to see a group of severely hunched-over elders in the television lounge. But when she came home that afternoon, Denise was shocked to realize that her teenage children and their friends slouched just the same way while they watched television.

Certainly age-related changes and conditions do occur. For example, as you get older the discs in your back lose some of their water content, becoming less spongy, more rigid, and narrower, exaggerating bad posture and stiffness. Hips and knees tend to become slightly more bent as you age, leading to walking pattern alterations. The possibility of developing conditions such as osteoporosis and spinal stenosis also increases with age. You can't turn back the hands of time. But with proper exercise and training, you can maintain and improve your body's performance despite advancing age.

ANATOMICAL AND HEALTH INFORMATION

Human Skeleton

The human skeleton is made up of a framework of 206 bones that act as the main structural support for the body. They protect the inner organs and serve as the primary attachments for most of the body's muscles. Red blood cells are created within bone marrow and bones and store necessary elements such as calcium, phosphorus, magnesium, and sodium. Strong bones are essential. To keep them strong, exercises (especially strengthening and weight-bearing exercises) must be a regular part of daily activity. Figure 2.1 provides a view of the human skeletal system.

When you look at the normal spine from the side, you can see 3 gentle front-to-back curves: frontward curves in the neck and lower back and a backward curve in the upper back. However, the normal spine appears straight when viewed from the back (Figure 2.2).

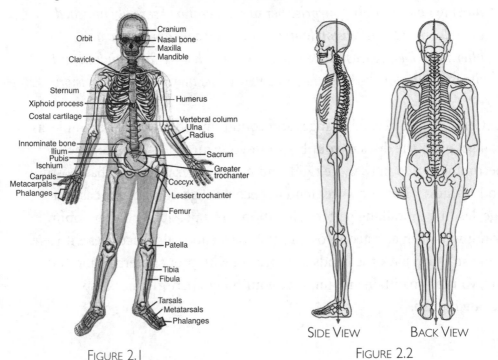

FIGURE 2.1   SIDE VIEW   BACK VIEW

FIGURE 2.2

What the Research Has To Say About Osteoporosis

Numerous studies have shown the effectiveness of exercise on improving bone mineral density (BMD), also called bone density. Some of these studies and their findings are summarized below.

An article published in the *Annals of Internal Medicine* reported that women who had higher activity levels (sports, housework, and leisure time) had a 36 percent reduction in the incidence of hip fractures.

An article in the *Journal of the American Medical Association* demonstrated that high-intensity strength training is an effective and feasible means to preserve bone density while improving muscle mass, strength, and balance in postmenopausal women.

An article in the *Mayo Clinic Proceedings* showed that stronger back muscles decrease the incidence of vertebral fractures.

An article in *The Lancet* showed that high-impact exercise (exercise that loads bones with a rapidly rising force) improves BMD, muscle strength, and balance with no increased risk of fracture.

An article in the *American Journal of Physical Medicine and Rehabilitation* demonstrated how a senior dance program significantly improved BMD, compared to a group who did not participate in the program.

Finally, an article in the *Journal of Gerontology* presented a meta-analysis, a thorough investigation of numerous studies on osteoporosis; it found that exercise improves BMD in the back.

Chart I
OSTEOPOROSIS EVALUATION SCORE SHEET

1. **What is your current age?** [ ] Years   Multiply the number in
   the shaded block by 3
   and enter

   _____

2. **What is your race or ethnic group?** (Check one)
   Black ❑   Enter 0
   White ❑ Hispanic ❑ Asian ❑   Enter 5
   Native American/American Indian ❑   Enter 5
   Other ❑   Enter 5

   _____

3. **Have you ever been treated for or told you have
   rheumatoid arthritis?**
   Yes ❑ No ❑   If yes, enter 4

   _____

4. **Since the age of 45, have you experienced a fracture
   (broken bone) at any of the following sites?**
   Hip   Yes ❑   No ❑   If yes, enter 4
   Rib   Yes ❑   No ❑   If yes, enter 4
   Wrist Yes ❑   No ❑   If yes, enter 4

   _____
   _____

5. **Do you currently take or have you ever taken medicine
   containing estrogen?** (Examples include Premarin, Estrace,
   Estraderm, and Estratab.)
   Yes ❑ No ❑   If no, enter 1

   _____

   Add score from questions 1–5.

   Subtotal

6. **What is your current weight?** [ ] lbs   Enter the two numbers
   in the shaded blocks and
   subtract this number
   from Subtotal

   _____

   FINAL
   SCORE

   **IF YOUR FINAL SCORE IS 6 OR HIGHER, YOU SHOULD BE EVALUATED
   FURTHER FOR OSTEOPOROSIS. TALK TO YOUR DOCTOR.**

Health-related conditions

Osteoporosis, scoliosis, and spinal stenosis are conditions that affect posture and require consultation with a healthcare professional. If you have been diagnosed with one of these conditions, a program of increasing physical conditioning, along with appropriate treatment, will enhance your fitness and functional ability.

Osteoporosis is an excessive loss of bone density that causes porous and fragile bones. A person with osteoporosis can break bones such as the hip, spine, or wrist in falls even during daily activities. For example, a woman with severe osteoporosis might fracture a bone in her spine simply by attempting to raise a stuck window. Osteoporosis affects 28 million people in the United States, and women are affected 4 times more often than men. One in 2 women will experience an osteoporosis-related fracture sometime in her lifetime; only 1 in 8 men will.

Often people show no signs or symptoms of osteoporosis until a fracture occurs. Chart 1 (page 28) is an evaluation score sheet that will help you determine if you are at high risk for osteoporosis. If your score is higher than 6, consult a physician. He or she may suggest a bone density assessment, an easy, painless measure of the body's ability to absorb radiation (called absorptiometry or tomography) or sound waves (called ultrasound). If you have experienced bone loss, your physician will recommend a course of treatment that may include exercise, calcium and vitamin D supplements, and medication.

Scoliosis is a side-to-side curvature of the spine affecting about 4 percent of the U.S. population: 1 in 9 females and a smaller percentage of men. Figure 2.3a depicts the normal spine alignment as viewed from the front or back and 2.3b depicts the side-to-side curavture of scoliosis from the front or back.

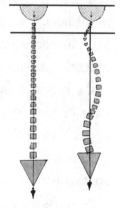

FIGURE 2.3A   2.3B

A very mild scoliosis may not cause problems, but a more significant curvature may result in muscle imbalance, weakness, and fatigue, and may lead to more severe problems, such as major spinal changes and breathing difficulty.

To test yourself for scoliosis, stand barefoot in your underwear in front of a full-length mirror. See if the center of your nose, chin, breastbone, and belly button appear to be in a fairly straight line. Let your arms hang down at your sides; the distance between your arms and your body should be similar on each side. Now place your hands on the top of your pelvic bones with your fingers pointing forward; you hands should be level; so should your shoulders. If you suspect you have scoliosis, consult a physician and physical therapist.

Spinal stenosis is the result of the following possible changes in the spine: 1) a narrowing of the canal through which the spinal cord passes; 2) a narrowing of the pathways through which the nerves pass; or 3) a narrowing of the openings between two vertebrae. Stenosis may occur in either the lumbar or cervical spine areas, but is much more common in the lumbar spine. It is an increasingly common cause of lower back and leg pain in persons over 55 because the likelihood of developing lumbar spinal stenosis increases with age, especially in today's population of active, long-living adults. Pressure on the nerves may lead to a sensation of numbness, tingling, or brief periods of muscle weakness. Pain resulting from lumbar spinal stenosis can begin in the back and run through the buttocks and into the thigh, leg, and foot. It usually lessens when sitting and increases when arching the back, standing, or walking. Pain resulting from cervical spinal stenosis can begin in the neck and run down the upper arm in the forearm and fingers.

One simple test for lumbar spinal stenosis is to stand, arch your back as far as possible, hold the position for 30 seconds, and note if any of the symptoms occur. Other tests may be done by a healthcare professional to see if spinal stenosis or something else is the underlying cause of back-related problems. A definite diagnosis must be based on objective examinations such as magnetic resonance imaging techniques (MRI). The treatment for stenosis in the lumbar spine varies from exercises and adjustments in postural alignment during daily activities to bracing and surgery. The treatment for stenosis in the cervical spine varies from exercise and adjustments in postural alignment during daily activities to use of a collar, special cervical pillow, and surgery.

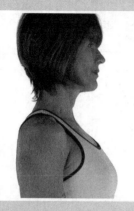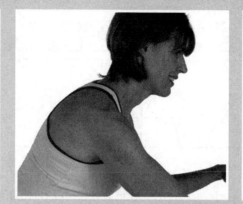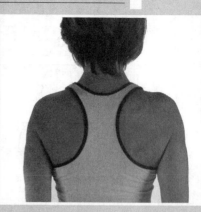

POSTURE ASSESSMENT

The following assessment will help you judge your posture. Take each test as described and record your results. After completing the tests, use the checklist to create your own posture profile and develop your most effective exercise program. Remember that most bodies are not perfectly symmetrical, so small deviations are normal.

For the most accurate assessment of your posture, have someone look at you and grade you from the side, front, and back. Perhaps you and a friend could evaluate each other. If this is not possible, you may do a self-assessment in front of a full-length, three-way mirror looking from the side and front. Deviations should be graded by severity as indicated on the checklist. In addition, note the direction of the deviation. For example, if your head tilts, note this on the form.

Additional spaces are provided so that you can evaluate yourself again after you have performed the exercises for 8 weeks.

HEAD

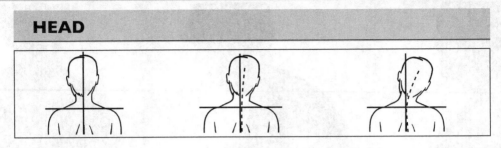

Action: To test the alignment of your head, stand facing the mirror or a friend. Imagine a line that runs perpendicular to the floor. The center of your forehead should be in line with your nose, the middle of your chin, and the middle of the upper part of your breastbone.

Score:

- If the imaginary line passes directly through the center of your head, give yourself a 10.

- If your head turns or tilts slightly in relation to the line, give yourself a 5.

- If your head is turned or tilted markedly, give yourself a 0.

Score:	Score:	Score:
Date:	Date:	Date:

Assessment: If your score is 5 or 0, do exercise 4. A low score on head alignment is easily fixed, so following recommendations will soon deliver positive results.

SHOULDERS

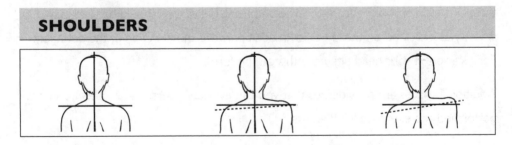

Action: To test the alignment of your shoulders, stand facing the mirror or a friend.

Score:

- If your shoulders are level, give yourself a 10.

- If one shoulder is slightly higher than the other, give yourself a 5.

- If one shoulder is significantly higher than the other, give yourself a 0.

Score:	Score:	Score:
Date:	Date:	Date:

Assessment: If your score is 5 or 0, do exercises 1 and 4. You don't want to look and feel lopsided! Commit to these exercises for 2 months. You'll soon see a difference in the mirror.

SPINE

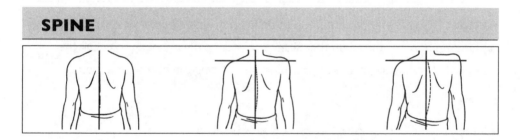

Action: To test the alignment of your spine, stand face a 3-way mirror or a friend. View your spine from the back and then from the front. From the back, the middle of your skull, the bones of your back, and the cleft of your buttocks should be in a straight line; from the front, the center of your breast bone and belly button should be in a straight line.

Score:

- If there's no curvature in your spine, give yourself a 10.

- If you note a slight curve, give yourself a 5.

- If you see a distinct curve, give yourself a 0.

Score:	Score:	Score:
Date:	Date:	Date:

Assessment: If your score is 5 or 0, do exercises 1, 7, and 8. Too much of a spine curvature (indicated by a low score) can cause future muscle imbalance. If you recognize and attend to this problem early, you can prevent potentially serious problems.

HIPS

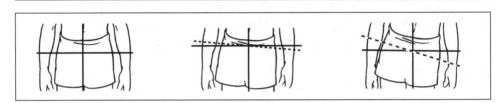

Action: This test is important because your body works better when it is symmetrical. Uneven hips can throw off the balance of your spine and neck, so check this carefully. To test the alignment of your hips, stand facing the mirror or a friend.

Score:

- If the height of both hips is the same, give yourself a 10.

- If one hip is slightly higher than the other, give yourself a 5.

- If one hip is markedly higher than the other, give yourself a 0.

Score:	Score:	Score:
Date:	Date:	Date:

Assessment: If your score is 5 or 0, do exercises 2 and 3.

NECK

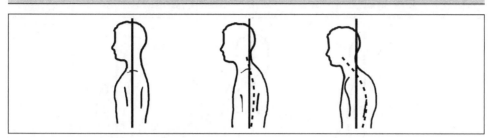

Action: The best way to test the alignment of your neck is to have a friend observe you from the side. If this is not possible, stand sideways in front of the mirror; try not to turn while you observe yourself.

Score:

- If your neck is erect, your chin in, and your earlobe directly above your shoulder, give yourself a 10.

- If your neck is slightly forward and your chin is slightly out, give yourself a 5.

- If your neck is markedly forward and your chin is noticeably out, give yourself a 0.

Score:	Score:	Score:
Date:	Date:	Date:

Assessment: If your score is 5 or 0, do exercises 1 and 8. Postural alignment begins with the head, so the correct neck position is extremely important.

UPPER BACK

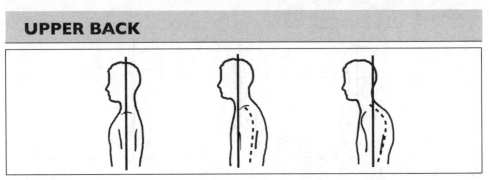

Action: The best way to test the alignment of your upper back is to have a friend observe you from the side. If this is not possible, stand sideways in front of the mirror; try not to turn while you observe yourself.

Score:

- If you see a slight, gentle rounding of your back, give yourself a 10.

- If you see moderate rounding of your upper back, give yourself a 5.

- If you see an obvious rounding of your upper back, give yourself a 0.

Score:	Score:	Score:
Date:	Date:	Date:

Assessment: If your score is 5 or 0, do exercises 5, 6, and 8. Problems with upper body posture are often associated with the forward head position described in the Neck section. Plus, if you scored low on Head you may also score low on this test. If so, you really need to do these exercises, especially if you tend to assume this posture without thinking. These exercises may be difficult at first, but they can be done. Once you have mastered them, you will find breathing and movement so much easier.

ABDOMEN

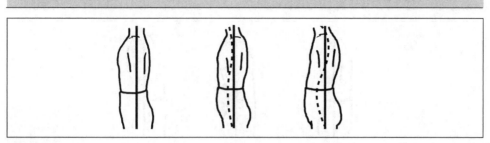

Action: This is our least favorite evaluation. It is best to observe yourself, since it isn't pleasant to have someone else tell you that you have a sagging, protruding abdomen. The good news is that with exercise you can have a flatter, tighter stomach. Stand sideways in front of the mirror; try not to turn while you observe yourself.

Score:

- If your abdomen is flat, give yourself a 10.

- If your abdomen protrudes slightly, give yourself a 5.

- If your abdomen protrudes significantly, give yourself a 0.

Score:	Score:	Score:
Date:	Date:	Date:

Assessment:

- If your score is 5 or 0, do exercises 1 and 8 and also see the exercises for Trunk Flexion in chapter 3.

LOWER BACK

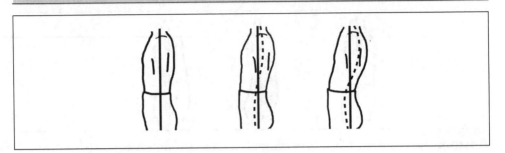

Action: This is a very important area and a pivotal point in any physical therapy or orthopedic exam. The hollowing of the back may indicate back problems. Carefully do this test and strictly follow the exercises suggested. The best way to test the alignment of your lower back is to have a friend observe you from the side. If this is not possible, stand sideways in front of the mirror; try not to turn while you observe yourself.

Score:

■ If there is a gentle curve in your lower back, give yourself a 10.

■ If there is a moderate hollowing in your lower back, give yourself a 5.

■ If there is a marked hollowing, give yourself a 0.

Assessment: If your score is 5 or 0, do exercises 1 and 8.

Score:	Score:	Score:
Date:	Date:	Date:

TOTAL SCORE

Add up your results from all the tests. A perfect score is 80. Based on our many years of practice, we would have to say that less than 5 percent of the population achieves perfection.

If your total score is below 40 or if you get a 0 in any one area, consider getting a thorough assessment by a physical therapist. Don't be alarmed—just know that you may need some extra help to get started on these exercises. If your muscles and joints are especially tight, they may need physical therapy techniques such as mobilization and soft-tissue work or modalities (heat, ultrasound, electrical stimulation) to loosen them so that these exercises can be more effective.

A score of 5 in any area could be cause for concern, but you can improve your results using the exercises in this chapter. Our clients and patients tell us how simple but amazing these exercises are; they get results. Be patient initially. You may notice a difference in a short time, but you will probably need to continue the exercises for a few weeks to see significant results. Take the tests again after doing the exercises for 2 months and see if your scores have improved.

Wendy's Prescription for Posture

Wendy scored a 65 on the Posture Score Sheet. She received scores of 5 in Neck, Upper Back, and Abdomen. To improve these areas, she decided to perform Pelvic Tilt and Axial Extensions (exercise 1), Isometric Elbow Press Backs (exercise 5), Pectoral Stretches (exercise 6), and "W" Wall Stretches with Knee Bend (exercise 8) every day for 2 months.

James's Prescription for Posture

James scored a 40 on the Posture Score Sheet, receiving 5 in each posture area. Since he needed work in so many areas, he decided to do all of the exercises in this chapter every day for 2 months.

PRESCRIPTION FOR POSTURE

Date: _____

Head　　　　Score: _____ Exercise(s) Needed:_____

Shoulders　Score: _____ Exercise(s) Needed:_____

Spine　　　Score: _____ Exercise(s) Needed:_____

Hips　　　　Score: _____ Exercise(s) Needed:_____

Neck　　　　Score: _____ Exercise(s) Needed:_____

Upper Back　Score: _____ Exercise(s) Needed:_____

Abdomen　　Score: _____ Exercise(s) Needed:_____

Lower Back　Score: _____ Exercise(s) Needed:_____

(Make a copy for your personal use)

8 GREAT EXERCISES FOR POSTURE

#1 Pelvic Tilt and Axial Extensions

#2 Hip Flexor Stretches

#3 Hamstring Stretches

#4 Chin Tucks

#5 Isometric Elbow Press Backs

#6 Pectoral Stretches

#7 Wall Reaches

#8 "W" Wall Stretches with Knee Bends

#1 ■ Pelvic Tilt and Axial Extensions

Why this exercise? This exercise is a wonderful way to align your back and head and to help you stand straight. It is important to combat the daily stresses of sitting and standing that negatively impact spinal curves. While a slight spinal curve is natural and expected, too much of one can cause pain, stiffness, and difficulty moving during daily activities.

1. Lie on your back with your feet flat on the floor, your knees bent, and your arms outstretched. Breathe in (photo 1).

2. Tighten your stomach muscles, gently pinch your buttocks together, and pull in your chin so the back of your neck flattens as you breathe out (photo 2).

3. Hold this position for 10 seconds while you breathe deeply and relax.

4. Begin with 3 repetitions, gradually increasing to 10 or 20.

5. Perform this exercise once or twice a day.

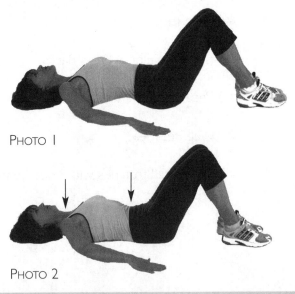

PHOTO 1

PHOTO 2

#2 ■ Hip Flexor Stretches

Why this exercise? Standing or walking unevenly puts stress on joints and muscles, resulting in discomfort and stiffness. If you tilt to the side when you stand, then
1 of your hips is probably higher than the other because the muscles on the other
side are tighter. This stretch will help loosen the tight muscles so that your hips are
level. Concentrate on the tight side by doing 3 repetitions of this exercise on that
side and only 1 on the other. Once your hip muscles are more symmetrical, you
will be able to stand evenly.

1. Lie on your back with your knees bent and your feet flat on the
floor. As you breathe in, pull in your stomach and chin so that your
neck and lower back flatten (photo 1).

2. Bring your right knee to your chest and wrap your hands under
your thigh as you breathe out.

3. Slowly slide your left leg down until it is flat against the floor. Hold
the position for 30 seconds as you breathe deeply. **Tip:** Count out
loud while exhaling to make sure you continue to breathe during the
hold (photo 2).

4. Return your left leg
and then your right
leg to the starting
position.

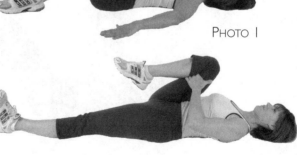

PHOTO 1

5. Repeat on the left
side.

6. Do 3 repetitions
for each leg, alternat-
ing sides, or begin by
concentrating on the
tighter side as noted above.

PHOTO 2

7. Perform this exercise once or twice a day.

#3 ■ Hamstring Stretches

Why this exercise? If 1 or both of your knees are bent when you stand, this stretch will help you stand straighter. If 1 knee is bent more than the other, then the muscles on 1 side are probably tighter. Concentrate on that side by doing 3 repetitions of this exercise on that side and only 1 on the other. Once your hamstring muscles are symmetrical, you will be able to stand straighter. Standing or walking unevenly can cause discomfort and stress.

1. Lie on your back with your knees bent and your feet flat on the floor. As you breathe in, pull in your stomach and chin so that your neck and lower back flatten (photo 1).

2. Straighten your left leg, keeping it below the level of your right knee as you breathe out.

3. Lock your left knee and pull your left foot up toward you, flexing your foot at the ankle (photo 2).

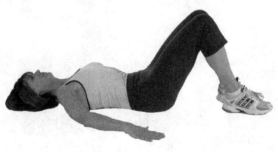

PHOTO 1

4. Raise your left leg as high as comfortably possible. Hold this position for 30 seconds as you breathe deeply (photo 2).

5. Bring your left leg back to the starting position.

6. Repeat, using your right leg.

7. Do 3 repetitions of this exercise on each side, alternating sides, or concentrating on the tighter side.

8. Perform this exercise once or twice a day.

Note: Place a towel (or belt or strap) around the foot of your extended leg to help increase the stretch (photo 3).

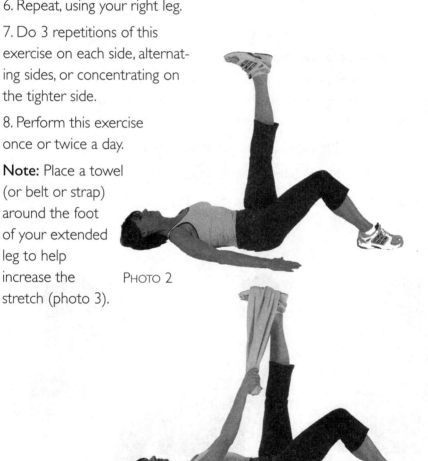

PHOTO 2

PHOTO 3

#4 ■ Chin Tucks

Why this exercise? This exercise is wonderful for improving a forward head position. The daily stresses of sitting and standing negatively impact the curve of the neck. While a slight spinal curve is natural and expected, too much curvature can cause pain, stiffness, and difficulty in moving during daily activities.

1. Sit in a supportive chair as erectly as you can (photo 1).

2. Keeping your head straight, breathe in and draw your head back so that your neck is in line with your spine (photo 2). **Tip:** If you have difficulty achieving this position, take your index finger, place it in the middle of your chin, and push your chin back and up (inset).

3. Hold this position for 10 seconds as you breathe deeply.

4. Repeat this exercise 5 times every hour.

5. **Note:** This exercise may also be done standing.

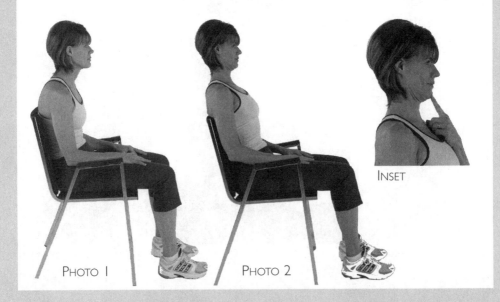

INSET

PHOTO 1   PHOTO 2

#5 ■ Isometric Elbow Press Backs

Why this exercise? This exercise is a terrific way to strengthen the neglected mid-back muscles. Because you mostly use your front chest muscles during daily activities, your mid-back muscles tend to become weak.

1. Sit in a supportive chair or stand against a wall. Tuck your chin in (photo 1). Breathe in.

2. Bend your elbows at your sides and close your fingers in a relaxed fist (photo 2).

3. Gently press your elbows back into the back of the chair or the wall (photo 3).

4. Hold this position for 10 seconds as you breathe deeply. Do not move.

5. Breathe in and release the position slowly.

6. Begin with 3 repetitions of this exercise and build to 10 or 20.

7. Perform this exercise once or twice a day.

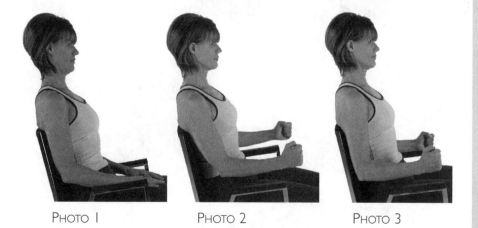

PHOTO 1   PHOTO 2   PHOTO 3

#6 ■ Pectoral Stretches

Why this exercise? Hours spent sitting and slumping can tighten your chest muscles. This simple stretch can help elongate these muscles, allowing you to stand straighter and breathe more easily because your chest can expand more freely. You'll need a cane or a broom handle for this exercise.

1. Lie on your back with your knees bent, your feet flat on the floor, and your arms at your side.

2. Holding a cane or broom handle in both hands, bend your elbows and raise your forearms so that your hands face the ceiling (photo 1).

3. Keeping your upper arms on the floor, slowly try to bring the cane or broom handle over your head and back toward the floor as you breathe out (photo 2).

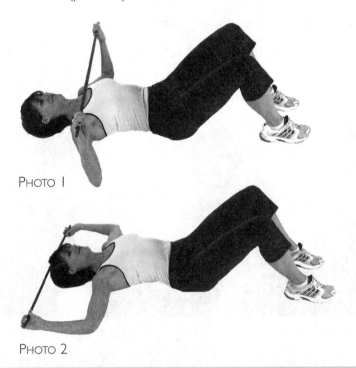

PHOTO 1

PHOTO 2

4. Hold this position without moving for 30 seconds, breathing deeply.

5. Slowly return the cane or broom handle to the starting position.

6. Do 3 repetitions of this exercise.

7. Perform this exercise once or twice a day.

Pectoral Stretch, Alternate Technique

1. Lie in the same position as above. Place your hands behind your head with your elbows facing up.

2. Keeping your hands behind your head, press your elbows to the floor as you breathe in (photo 4).

3. Hold this position for 30 seconds while breathing deeply.

4. Slowly return your arms to the starting position.

5. Do 3 repetitions of this exercise.

6. Perform once or twice a day.

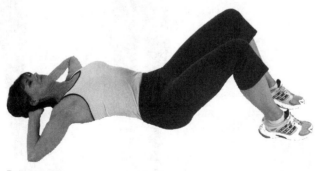

PHOTO 4

#7 ■ Wall Reaches

Why this exercise? This exercise is a wonderful way to align your back. The daily stresses of sitting and standing negatively impact the curves of your spine. While a slight spinal curve is natural and expected, too much can cause slouching and weakness.

1. Stand facing a wall with your feet about 2 inches from the wall and your feet hip-width apart (photo 1).

2. Pull in your stomach and tuck in your chin as you breathe in.

3. Stretch your arms up the wall as high as possible as you lengthen your spine (photo 2).

4. Hold this position for 30 seconds while breathing deeply.

5. Lower your arms and relax.

6. Do 3 repetitions of this exercise.

7. Perform this exercise once or twice a day.

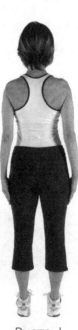

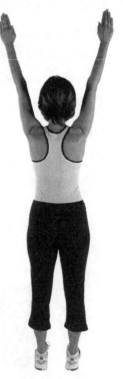

PHOTO 1   PHOTO 2

#8 ■ "W" Wall Stretches with Knee Bends

Why this exercise? This exercise is another good one to align your back and relieve pain, stiffness, and difficulty moving around during daily activities.

1. Stand with your back against a wall and your feet 18 to 24 inches from the wall and 6 to 8 inches apart.

2. Place your arms in a "W" position (photo 1).

3. Breathe in, pull in your stomach, and tuck in your chin while flattening your back and neck against the wall.

4. Breathe out while bending your knees about one-third of the way down, sliding your arms up the wall as high as possible, and lengthening your spine (photo 2). Try to keep your arms in contact with the wall as you slide them up.

5. Hold this position for 30 seconds while breathing deeply.

6. Lower your arms, straighten your knees, and relax.

7. Do 3 repetitions of this exercise.

8. Do this exercise once or twice a day.

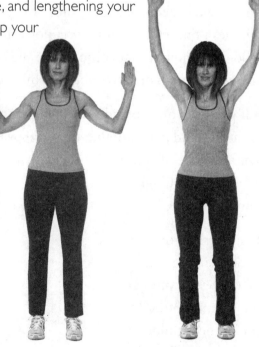

PHOTO 1   PHOTO 2

DAILY TIPS AND ENERGIZING IDEAS

This section includes easy-to-do tasks, modifications to daily activities, and hints to enhance and reinforce the exercises in your posture program. Place little notes to yourself everywhere you tend to look during the day as reminders to do them from time to time.

AT HOME

Sleeping

Selecting the correct pillow is important. Avoid large pillows that bend your neck too much—they can cause overstretching or tightening of neck muscles and ligaments. Foam pillows usually conform to the anatomical alignment of the neck, but they may not provide adequate support for your neck, tightening your muscles unnecessarily. A thicker polyester pillow or a contoured pillow of material that conforms to the curves of the neck (preferably memory foam) can enhance your neck alignment.

■ If you sleep on your side, use a pillow that keeps your head parallel to the bed and place another pillow between your knees (photo 1). The vertebrae of your neck should be in alignment with the rest of your spine, not higher or lower.

■ If you sleep on your back, use a contoured pillow (we recommend the Tempur-Pedic® or similar neck pillow) to keep your neck well aligned and place

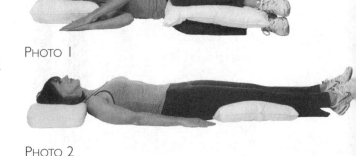

PHOTO I

PHOTO 2

another pillow under your knees if you
do not have any knee problems (photo 2).

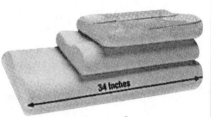

■ Avoid sleeping on your stomach, which
stresses the neck by overstretching some
muscles and tightening others.

TEMPUR-PEDIC® PILLOWS

Grooming

During all these activities, remember to keep your body as straight as
possible—stomach in and chin tucked.

■ While you brush your teeth, place your hand on the sink and
bend your knees
slightly (photo 3).

■ While you
shave or put on
makeup, stand up
straight (photo
4). Do not lean
toward the mir-
ror (photo 5). If
necessary, get a
mirror with an
extending arm to
bring the mirror
to your face.

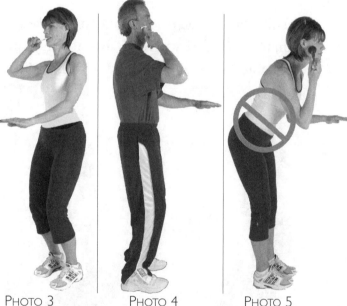

PHOTO 3   PHOTO 4   PHOTO 5

■ While dressing, keep your head and upper back well aligned, bend
from the hips and knees to keep your trunk straight, and always
remember to keep your stomach in and chin tucked.

■ While dressing, sit down rather than trying to balance awkwardly on one leg.

Preparing Meals

■ When you wash dishes, open the cabinet under the sink and place a foot on the bottom shelf (photo 6). Alternate feet every so often.

■ When you get things from lower shelves, bend your knees and keep your body well aligned (photo 7).

■ Store pots and pans at waist height so that you are not reaching too high or bending too far over to get them.

■ Think before you reach. Remember to keep your stomach in and chin tucked before you reach forward and upward. If an object is too high, use a stool (photo 8).

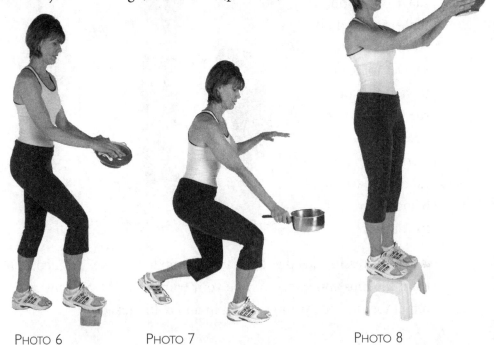

PHOTO 6   PHOTO 7   PHOTO 8

Showering

The shower is a great place to practice good posture.

■ Roll your shoulders and lengthen your spine.

■ Tuck in your chin and tighten your stomach.

■ Tilt your head side to side toward your shoulders; turn your head to the right and left.

■ Let your chin drop gently to your chest and roll your chin from side to side along your chest.

■ Stretch as tall as you can.

■ Let the warm water relax stressed body parts.

Sitting While Watching TV or Eating

■ Sit in a chair with good support. Avoid soft sofas, overstuffed couches, or chairs with pillows, which can lead to slumping and overstretching of joints and muscles.

■ Sit erect.

■ Perform a pelvic tilt every half hour. Pull your stomach in and gently squeeze your buttocks together while pressing your lower back into the back of your chair. Release.

■ Place a small stool (6 to 8 inches in height) under your feet to raise your knees slightly higher than your hips. This will help open and relax your back muscles, especially if you have spinal stenosis.

Standing

■ When you stand for a few moments (such as waiting for an elevator or for someone to pick you up), lean back against the wall with your feet about 6 inches away. Put your head against the wall and flatten your neck as much as possible. Feel the edges of your shoulder blades and bring them back and slightly downward. Notice how much straighter you are standing. Hold this position for 30 seconds and repeat several times while you are waiting.

ON YOUR WAY TO WORK

Driving

■ Maintain good posture. Move the seat forward so your knees are slightly higher than your hips (photo 9). To support your spine, place a small contoured pillow behind your lower back. The seat should be upright so that the headrest truly rests your head. Use the headrest as a support to do chin tucks when you are stopped in traffic.

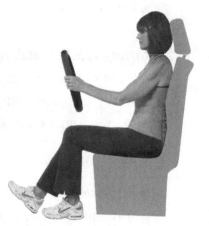

Walking

■ Be careful of what you carry. Heavy   PHOTO 9
briefcases or shoulder bags may hinder
good posture, cause muscles to contract unequally, and result in neck and back problems.

■ Use a backpack or two small, lightweight cases of equal weight, one on each shoulder or in each hand.

■ Be sure to keep your stomach in and your chin tucked as you walk so that you are well aligned.

AT WORK

■ Your office chair should allow good postural alignment. Your feet should easily touch the floor when your hips are all the way back in your chair (photo 10). You should not have to crane your neck to work. Arrange your workspace so you can work with your chin in the erect and tucked position.

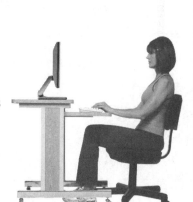

■ Your chair and workstation should encourage symmetry. For example, if you are always turning your head to the right, rearrange the space so you turn evenly in both directions. At the computer, your arms should be at your sides with your elbows bent and your wrists in neutral position. Your chin should be in, and you should look slightly down at your screen (photo 11).

PHOTO 10

■ Do chin tucks and seated pectoral stretches every hour.

■ If your work is sedentary, get up every half hour to do wall stretches, shrug your shoulders up and down, and roll your shoulders

PHOTO 11

back and forth. Also do this exercise every hour: stand up straight, tuck in your chin, bring your shoulders back and down, and tighten your stomach.

IN THE GYM

Gym equipment is often not meant for postural work. However, if you practice good alignment while exercising, it can lead to a powerful workout.

■ Always sit or stand straight while working out.

■ Tuck in your chin, bring your shoulders back and down, and tighten your stomach while using exercise equipment.

■ Place your feet on a small stool when using seated arm machines.

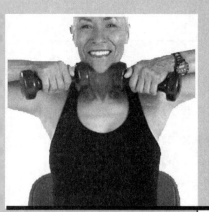

Chapter 3

Strength

Is Strength Training Safe?

Based on the research, the answer is a resounding "Yes!" Various studies have found that strength training can safely increase mobility for people of all ages. It is also beneficial for those with high blood pressure and cardiovascular disease.

So yes, strength training is safe—once you've had a thorough physical examination and learned the principles of safe resistance training. Before beginning a program, be sure that you are thoroughly familiar with all of our tips for using weights and the key points of the strengthening exercises (pages 86-88).

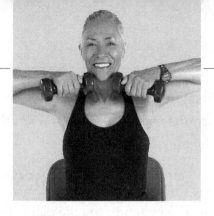

The older you get, the stronger the wind gets,
and it is always in your face.

—Jack Nicklaus

Strength is a key component of healthy physical performance; strong muscles help you move easily and enjoy life. And unlike many other things in life, muscles respond to stress in a positive way. They get stronger. Strength training is a safe and effective way to improve muscle capabilities and to increase healthy physical performance. Good programs do much more than add bulk—they help to sculpt and stabilize the body. You can gain strength and muscle size throughout your life. It is never too late to start.

PROPER STRENGTH

Strength is a muscle's ability to produce force or do work, such as lift a weight or climb a stair. Generally, the larger the muscle, the greater its ability to produce force. For example, the large muscles of the buttocks and the fronts of the thighs are naturally stronger than those in the forearm or the eye. Muscles develop the most between birth and adolescence and generally peak in strength in the thirties, but with regular strength training, they can continue to perform at increasing levels despite advancing age.

Diane, 54, didn't think of herself as old and weak while working at her bank job or performing her weekly chores, including grocery shopping and rolling out the trash can on pickup day. But when her eagerly awaited first grandchild was born, and within 6 months weighed 20 pounds, she found herself huffing and puffing after a few minutes of carrying the infant.

STRENGTH CHANGES

Muscle contraction allows action to take place. The action can be large (swinging a golf club), small (blinking), or static (standing still). As you age, your muscles tend to lose their ability to contract at a strong and efficient level. Atrophy (a reduction in muscle size) also occurs and may lead to decreased range of motion and loss of muscle bulk, particularly in the forearms, hands, lower legs, and feet. Between the ages of 30 and 80, most people experience a decline in physical strength of approximately 30 percent. Everyone has to do more to maintain and increase strength as they get older.

Strength loss associated with aging usually occurs almost imperceptibly and often goes unnoticed until normal activities—such as walking upstairs, carrying groceries, or picking up a grandchild—become arduous. All too often, when these tasks become more difficult, you do less. Decreased activity means your muscles are taxed less, and—somewhat perversely—your body adjusts to a lower level of activity. The result is that you gradually become weaker. But it doesn't have to be that way.

The truth is, no one at any age can take strength for granted. Whether you're moving from your late twenties to early thirties or from your sixties to your seventies, it's important to do a little more each day to avoid generalized weakness. With training, your muscles can continue to serve you well, even increasing in strength despite advancing age. In our offices we see many people who mistakenly believe that there is nothing they can do to get stronger as they get older; they believe that they just have to learn to live with being weaker. Not so! Research offers numerous examples of people from 40 to 100 years of age who—on a prescribed and monitored individual exercise program much like the one in this chapter—experience tremendous increases in strength. We delight in telling our clients and patients about a study that included only men and women over 90; after 6 weeks on an exercise plan, they achieved an almost 200 percent increase in strength.

ANATOMICAL AND HEALTH INFORMATION
Muscles

Muscles are the power behind movement. Attached to bones, usually by tendons, they contract in 3 ways—by shortening (bending your elbow to look at your watch), by maintaining consistent tension without movement (keeping your head upright), or by lengthening (walking down stairs).

Approximately 100 different muscles are found within the body in 3 major classifications: smooth, cardiac, and skeletal. Smooth muscles, over which you have no voluntary control, are found primarily within the internal organs (blood vessel walls, digestive tract, bladder). Cardiac muscle is also involuntary. This specialized type of muscle enables your heart to beat and pump blood throughout your body.

Skeletal muscles are the only ones over which you have conscious control; they enable you to move your body (see Figures 3.1 and 3.2 for front and back views of some of the skeletal

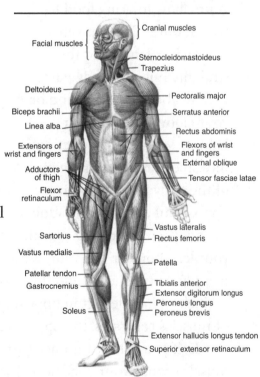

FIGURE 3.1

muscles). These are the muscles on which you concentrate in order to increase your strength.

Skeletal muscles affect all types of movement, including flexion, extension, abduction, adduction, and rotation. Flexion is the bending of a body part: your knees to squat or your elbow to bring food to your mouth. The opposite of flexion is extension or the straightening of a body part, such as your knees to stand or your elbow to lower your hand to your side. Abduction is movement away from the middle

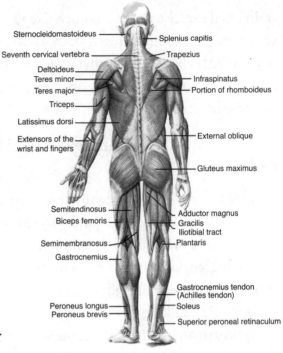

FIGURE 3.2

of the body: pushing your leg or raising your arm to the side. The opposite of abduction is adduction, or movement toward the middle of the body: crossing 1 leg over the other or bringing your right arm to your left shoulder. Rotation is movement around a pivot: turning the palm of your hand up and down or turning your head side to side.

Skeletal muscles act in opposing groups so that if 1 muscle or group of muscles contracts, the opposing muscle or group relaxes. In other words, if you bend your knee (using your hamstrings), the opposing muscle group (your quadriceps) will relax.

Skeletal muscles are composed of 2 types of fibers. Type I, called slow-twitch fibers, enhance endurance, helping to sustain muscle activity over long periods of time. They are best trained with a high number of repetitions and low weight. Type II, or fast-twitch fibers, enable rapid movement for performing quick, short bursts of activity and should be trained with fewer repetitions and heavier weights. Abdominal muscles are almost exclusively made up of Type I fibers, so to strengthen them, you should perform many repetitions of a partial sit up, using no or very low weights. Thigh muscles are composed mostly of Type II fibers, so to strengthen them, you would use heavier weights and fewer repetitions.

The 3 major types of muscle contractions are isometric, isotonic, and eccentric. An isometric contraction occurs when a muscle contracts and produces force but no movement. When you press your palms together, the muscles of your arms and chest are contracting even though your hands aren't moving. An isotonic contraction causes movement through an arc of motion, such as lifting your leg as you climb a step or raising your knee toward your chest when you sit down. An eccentric contraction occurs when a muscle acts as a brake to control weight as the muscle is lengthened. When you squat slowly, your front thigh muscles perform eccentric contractions. Eccentric contractions may be associated with muscle soreness.

Health-related Conditions

Strength can be affected by a number of conditions, including disease, inactivity, and failure to exercise correctly or often enough. Muscle spasms, strains, and tears can also cause problems. Muscles subjected to repetitive stress can weaken. Arthritis may cause muscle spasms and, in some cases, weakness.

A *muscle spasm* is the sudden and involuntary contraction of a muscle or group of muscles. If your body experiences a trauma (for example, whiplash, an injury to the back as a result of lifting a heavy object, or a twisted knee in a fall), it immediately tries to protect the injured part by keeping it still. The muscle goes into spasm to keep itself immobile. Relaxation of the spasm is necessary before treatment of the injury can begin.

A *strain* is a stress or overstretching of fibers that results in sore, painful, and sometimes stiff muscles. A strain may also cause tearing of the blood vessels within the muscle, leading to increased inflammation and possibly muscle spasm. Runners and other athletes may be prone to strains (and even small muscle tears) if they do not appropriately warm up or stretch. If you sharply increase your activity after being sedentary for a while, you may strain a muscle. PRICE therapy—Protection, Rest, Ice, Compression, and Elevation of the affected muscle—helps alleviate a strain during the first few days. Muscle strength will gradually return as the pain subsides.

A *tear* may be the result of a major trauma to a muscle or a longstanding impingement syndrome (see below). While any muscle may tear, this injury most frequently occurs in the muscles of the thigh (quadriceps and hamstrings), calf (gastrocnemius), and shoulder rotator cuff (especially the supraspinatus). Depending upon the severity of the injury, muscle tears may be treated with bracing or other support devices; physical therapy may also be used for pain control and muscle strengthening. If the tear is complete, surgery may be necessary.

Repetitive motions can lead to overuse and thus to *impingement syndrome,* the result of excessive friction between the joint tissues. This often occurs in the shoulder joint. Due to their anatomy, the muscles of the rotator cuff are prone to friction or unwanted compression of the joint tissue, particularly from repeated overhead activities such as serving a tennis ball or painting a ceiling. Symptoms may include pain and weakness in the surrounding muscles and increased difficulty with daily activities involving use of the muscle. Treatment usually involves special types of massage, strengthening exercises, and muscle retraining to eliminate the cause of the problem.

Both *osteoarthritis* and *rheumatoid arthritis* may result in muscle problems. Osteoarthritis, a degenerative joint disease that affects over 16 million people in the United States, may appear without symptoms in people as young as 30. Osteoarthritis occurs equally in men and women before the age of 55, but after that the incidence is higher in women. Rheumatoid arthritis, a chronic joint disease that affects over 2 million people in the United States, may be the result of a bacterial or viral infection or may be related to an autoimmune system disorder. It may occur at any age, though the peak incidence is between the ages of 25 and 55 years and is also found in older people. Women are affected two and a half times more than men.

Both disorders may produce painful, swollen, and stiff joints, though the extent of muscle involvement is more severe with rheumatoid arthritis. Muscles around arthritic joints may spasm, resulting in pain and an inability to move, and the disease may cause a decrease in muscle size that leads to wasting. Treatment programs for arthritis include pain control, joint motion enhancement, and muscle strengthening.

MUSCLE CAPABILITY

Different muscles have varying strength abilities, often as a result of how they are used and how much demand is placed upon them. These 3 experiments provide insight into the differences in muscle capabilities:

Hold a book. Stand up. Hold a heavy book (about 5 pounds) in front of you at chest height, keeping your arms straight (photo 1). Hold it there for 2 minutes. Most people will find this difficult unless they have been engaged in an upper-arm strengthening program. That is because the anterior deltoid muscles at the

PHOTO I

very front of the shoulder are doing most of the work. These relatively small muscles are usually only involved in motion, not holding.

Stand tall. Tuck in your chin as described in the Posture chapter (photo 2). Hold this position for 3 minutes. Most people will be able to do this, but it probably will not feel easy or natural. Strengthening your postural muscles will make holding this position easier.

Sit against a wall. Stand with your back against a wall and your feet 18 to 24 inches away and 6 to 8 inches apart. Slide down the wall, bending your knees so that they are directly over or slightly behind your ankles (photo 3). Hold this position for 10 to 30 seconds. Return to standing. Do the muscles in the front of your thighs feel shaky? Maybe. But you were able to complete the wall slide because your leg muscles kept you in position. They are capable of responding to increased loads; that is what they do during walking and stair climbing.

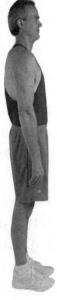
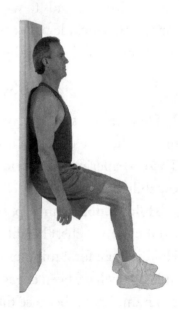

PHOTO 2   PHOTO 3

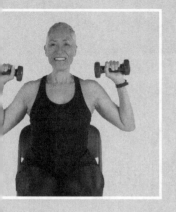
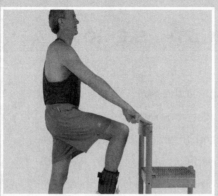

STRENGTH ASSESSMENT

The following assessment will help you judge the strength of your various muscles or muscle groups. Take each test as described and record your results. After completing the tests, use the checklist to create your own strength profile and develop your most effective exercise program. If you are concerned about particular strength deficits, we strongly suggest that you get a thorough muscle examination by a physical therapist who can tailor an effective program for you.

To perform these tests, you'll need an armless chair with good spine support, a stopwatch or clock with a second hand, and a 12-inch ruler. Wear sneakers or other flat shoes. You will need to have someone assist you with measurements. Some tests also require the Thera-band® (see page xiii). Tie the ends of the band together tightly to make a 12-inch loop (photo 1). Women use this 12-inch loop. Men will need to fold this loop in half to make a doubled 6-inch loop (photo 2).

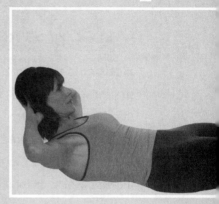

PHOTO 1

Think of these tests as fun. They'll help you see how strong you really are. Please don't overdo it or try to go beyond your limits.

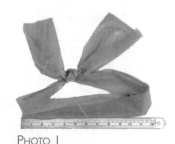

PHOTO 2

Additional spaces are available so that you can evaluate yourself again after you have performed the exercises for 8 weeks.

ELBOW STRENGTH: FLEXION

Action: To test your ability to bend your elbow, sit up straight with your back against the backrest of a chair. Put the Thera-band® loop under your right foot. Hold the other end in your right hand. (Men use doubled loop as explained on page 73.) Keep your arm at your side, with the elbow bent at approximately 90 degrees (photo 1). Slide your foot forward if you need to take up any slack. Bring your hand toward your shoulder as smoothly and slowly as you can, bending only your elbow. Do not arch your back to complete this test.

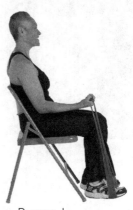

Photo 1

Have someone measure the length of the band when you have stretched it as far as comfortably possible. Repeat the test with your left arm.

Score: Record the distance you stretched the band on each side.

Right:	Right:	Right:
Left:	Left:	Left:
Date:	Date:	Date:

Assessment: Women should be able to stretch the band at least 28 inches. Men should be able to stretch the doubled band at least 15 inches. If you were unable to do so, do Arm exercise 6.

ELBOW STRENGTH: EXTENSION

Action: To test your ability to straighten your elbow, sit up straight with your back against the backrest of a chair. Place the Thera-band® loop under your right foot. Hold the other end in your right hand. (Men use doubled loop.) Lean forward so that

your chest is over your thighs.
Slide your foot forward if you
need to take up any slack.
With your left hand, hold
your right upper arm against
your side. Your right elbow
should be bent approximately
90 degrees (photo 1). Push
your right hand back as slowly

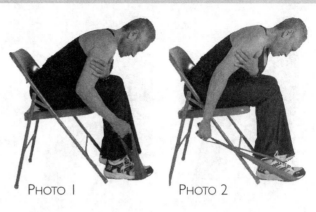

Photo 1   Photo 2

and smoothly as you can, straightening your elbow (photo 2).

Have someone measure the length of the band when you have stretched it as far as comfortably possible. Repeat the test with your left arm.

Score: Record the distance you stretched the band on each side.

Right:	Right:	Right:
Left:	Left:	Left:
Date:	Date:	Date:

Assessment: Women should be able to stretch the band at least 24 inches. Men should be able to stretch the doubled band at least 11 inches. If you were unable to do so, do Arm exercises 1 and 7.

SHOULDER STRENGTH: FLEXION

Action: To test your ability to raise your arm to the front, sit up straight with your back against the backrest of a chair. Let your right arm hang at your side with your palm facing the chair. Place the Thera-band® loop under your right foot. Hold the other end in your right hand (photo 1). (Men use doubled loop.) Slide your foot forward if you need to take up any slack. Raise your entire arm to the front while keeping your elbow straight (photo 2). Do not arch your back.

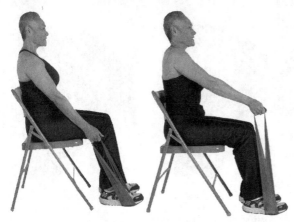

Have someone measure the length of the band when you have stretched it as far as comfortably possible. Repeat the test with your left arm.

Score: Record the distance you stretched the band on each side.

PHOTO I   PHOTO 2

Right:	Right:	Right:
Left:	Left:	Left:
Date:	Date:	Date:

Assessment: Women should be able to stretch the band at least 35 inches. Men should be able to stretch the doubled band at least 12 inches. If you were unable to do so, do Arm exercises 1, 2, and 4.

SHOULDER STRENGTH: ABDUCTION

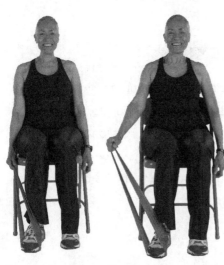

Action: To test your ability to raise your arm to the side, sit up straight with your back against the backrest of a chair. Let your right arm hang at your side with your palm facing the chair. Place the Thera-band® loop under your right foot. Hold the other end in your right hand (photo 1). (Men use doubled loop.) Slide your foot forward if you need to take up any slack. Raise your entire

PHOTO I   PHOTO 2

arm to the side, while keeping your elbow straight (photo 2). Do not lean to the opposite side to complete this test.

Have someone measure the length of the band when you have stretched it as far as comfortably possible. Repeat the test with your left arm.

Score: Record the distance you stretched the band on each side.

Right:	Right:	Right:
Left:	Left:	Left:
Date:	Date:	Date:

Assessment: Women should be able to stretch the band at least 30 inches. Men should be able to stretch the doubled band at least 8 inches. If you were unable to do so, do Arm exercise 5.

SHOULDER STRENGTH: EXTENSION

Action: To test your ability to raise your arm to the back, sit straight up with your back against the backrest of a chair. Let your right arm hang at your side with your palm facing the chair. Place the Thera-band® loop under your right foot. Hold the other end in your right hand (photo 1). (Men use doubled loop.) Slide your foot forward if you need to take up any slack. Push your entire arm backward, while keeping it straight (photo 2). Do not lean forward to complete this test.

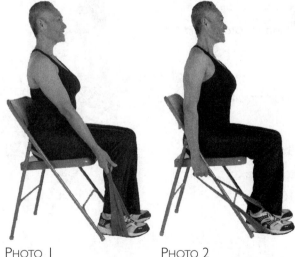

PHOTO 1   PHOTO 2

Have someone measure the length of the band when you have stretched it as far as comfortably possible. Repeat the test with your left arm.

Score: Record the distance you stretched the band on each side.

Right:	Right:	Right:
Left:	Left:	Left:
Date:	Date:	Date:

Assessment: Women should be able to stretch the band at least 32 inches. Men should be able to stretch the doubled band at least 11 inches. If you were unable to do so, do Arm exercise 8.

HIP AND KNEE STRENGTH: EXTENSION

Action: To test your ability to straighten your knees and stand, sit up straight in a chair. Do not lean back. Place your arms across your chest (photo 1). Using a stopwatch or a clock with a second hand, time yourself as you rise to a complete stand (photo 2) and return to a seated position 10 times in a row. Do not use your arms to complete this test.

Score: Record the time it took you to stand and sit 10 times.

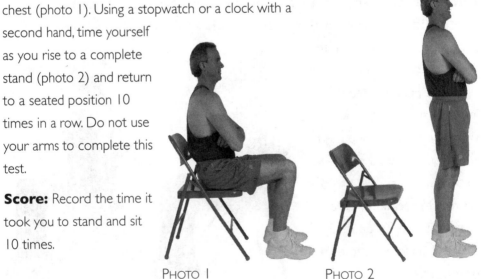

PHOTO 1   PHOTO 2

Score:	Score:	Score:
Date:	Date:	Date:

Assessment: Refer to Chart 1 in Chapter 1 (page 11). If your time is slower than the norm for your age and gender, do Leg exercises 1 and 5 and Neck and Trunk exercise 5.

HIP STRENGTH: ABDUCTION

Action: To test your ability to move your legs to the side, stand with the Thera-band® around your ankles (photo 1). Move your feet apart to take out any slack. (Men use doubled loop.) Place your arm against the wall for balance. Put your weight on your left leg. Slowly and smoothly lift your right leg out to the side, keeping it straight (photo 2).

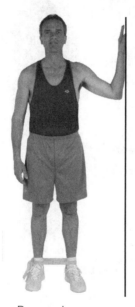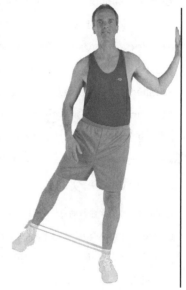

PHOTO 1   PHOTO 2

Have someone measure the length of the band when you have stretched it as far as comfortably possible. Repeat the test with your left leg.

Score: Record the distance you stretched the band on each side.

Right:	Right:	Right:
Left:	Left:	Left:
Date:	Date:	Date:

Assessment: Women should be able to stretch the band at least 30 inches. Men should be able to stretch the doubled band at least 12 inches. If you were unable to do so, do Leg exercise 3.

HIP STRENGTH: FLEXION

Action: To test your ability to flex your hips, twist the Thera-band® loop into a figure eight. (Men use doubled loop.) Place 1 loop around each foot (photo 1). Move your feet apart to take out any slack. Stand by a wall in case you need assistance balancing. Put your weight on your left leg. Raise your right knee toward your chest as high as comfortably possible (photo 2).

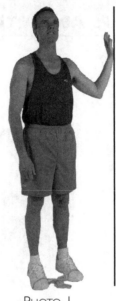 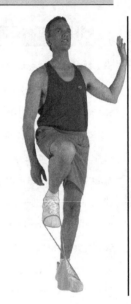

Have someone measure the length of the band when you have stretched it as far as comfortably possible. Repeat the test with your left leg.

PHOTO 1   PHOTO 2

Score: Record the distance you stretched the band on each side.

Right:	Right:	Right:
Left:	Left:	Left:
Date:	Date:	Date:

Assessment: Women should be able to stretch the band at least 20 inches. Men should be able to stretch the doubled band at least 13 inches. If you were unable to do so, do Leg exercises 2 and 4.

KNEE STRENGTH: FLEXION

Action: To test your ability to bend your knee, twist the Thera-band® loop into a figure 8. (Men use doubled loop.) Place 1 loop around your left foot and the other around your right ankle (photo 1). Move your feet apart to take out any slack. Stand by a wall in case you need assistance balancing. Put your weight on your left leg. Bend your right knee, raising your right foot as far up as possible (photo 2). Keep your thighs aligned and move only your lower leg.

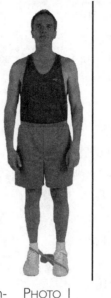
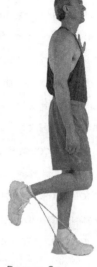

PHOTO 1   PHOTO 2

Have someone measure the length of the band when you have stretched it as far as comfortably possible. Repeat the test with your left leg.

Score: Record the distance you stretched the band on each side.

Right:	Right:	Right:
Left:	Left:	Left:
Date:	Date:	Date:

Assessment: Women should be able to stretch the band at least 20 inches. Men should be able to stretch the doubled band at least 13 inches. If you were unable to do so, do Leg exercise 6.

ANKLE AND TOE STRENGTH: FLEXION 1

Action: To test your ankle and toe strength, stand on your right leg and lift your left leg off the floor. Bend your left knee 90 degrees. If you have difficulty balancing, lightly place 1 or 2 fingers on a table, counter, or wall (photo 1). Slowly and smoothly, rise to your toes on your right foot (photo 2), and return to the starting position. Repeat 10 times or as many times as you can without discomfort.

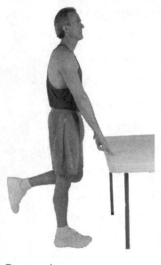

PHOTO 1

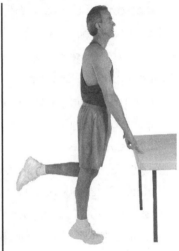

PHOTO 2

Repeat the test with your left leg.

Score: Record the number of times you were able to perform this movement on each leg.

Right:	Right:	Right:
Left:	Left:	Left:
Date:	Date:	Date:

Assessment: If you were unable to complete this movement 10 times on each side, do Leg exercise 7.

ANKLE AND TOE STRENGTH: FLEXION 2

Action: To test your ankle and toe strength, stand on your right leg and lift your left leg off the floor. Bend your left knee 90 degrees and your right knee about 45 degrees. If you have difficulty balancing, lightly place 1 or 2 fingers on a table, counter, or wall. Slowly and smoothly, rise to your toes on your right foot, keeping your knee bent (photo 1) and return to the starting position. Repeat 10 times or as many times as you can without discomfort.

Repeat the test with your left leg.

Score: Record the number of times you were able to perform the movement on each leg.

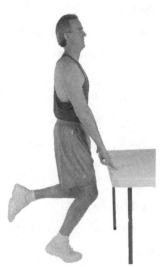

PHOTO 1

Right:	Right:	Right:
Left:	Left:	Left:
Date:	Date:	Date:

Assessment: : If you were unable to complete this movement 10 times, do Leg exercise 7.

ANKLE AND TOE STRENGTH: EXTENSION

Action: To test your ankle and toe strength, stand on your right leg and lift your left leg off the floor. Bend your left knee 90 degrees. If you have difficulty balancing, lightly place 1 or 2 fingers on a table, counter, or wall. Slowly and smoothly, raise the toes of your right foot up as much as possible and return to the starting position. Don't rock your foot, just lift your toes (photo 1). Repeat 5 times or as many times as you can without discomfort.

Repeat the test with your left leg.

Score: Record the number of times you are able to perform the movement on each leg.

Right:	Right:	Right:
Left:	Left:	Left:
Date:	Date:	Date:

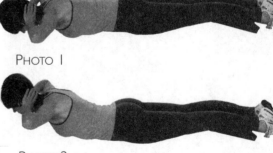

PHOTO 1

Assessment: If you are unable to complete this movement 5 times, do Leg exercise 8.

BACK STRENGTH: EXTENSION

Caution: If you are experiencing any back problems, consult your physician and physical therapist before performing this test.

PHOTO 1

Action: To test your ability to stand straight and arch your back, lie on your stomach with the tops of your feet flat on the floor. Clasp your hands behind your head

PHOTO 2

(photo 1). Keeping your feet flat on the floor, lift your head and upper trunk so that your chin is approximately 7 inches off the floor (photo 2).

Score: Have someone measure the distance between your chin and the floor.

Score:	Score:	Score:
Date:	Date:	Date:

Assessment: If you are unable to lift your head and upper trunk at least 7 inches off the floor, do Arm exercise 3 and Neck and Trunk exercises 6 and 7.

ABDOMINAL STRENGTH: FLEXION

Caution: If you have osteoporosis of your upper spine, consult your physician and physical therapist before performing this test.

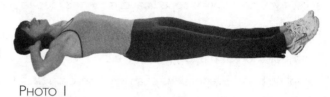

PHOTO 1

Action: To test your abdominal muscle strength, lie on your back with your legs straight. Clasp your hands behind your head

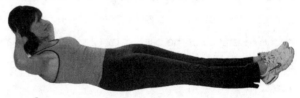

PHOTO 2

(photo 1) and tuck your chin into your chest. Using your abdominal muscles, smoothly lift your head and shoulders until your shoulder blades are just off the floor (photo 2). Keep your legs and feet on the floor. Do not pull up on your head with your hands.

Score: Have someone measure the distance between the highest point on the back of your shoulders and the floor.

Score:	Score:	Score:
Date:	Date:	Date:

Assessment: If you are unable to lift your shoulder blades off the floor, do Neck and Trunk exercises 1, 2, 3, 4, and 8.

HOW MUCH WEIGHT SHOULD I LIFT?

Before you begin a strength training program, you need to know how much weight you can and should lift. Physical therapists have various techniques to assess their clients' and patients' abilities, but you can easily perform this alternate evaluation at home using hand and cuff weights or a Thera-band®. It's a process of trial and error. Start with a low weight. (If you are using the Thera-band®, you have 2 options. You can purchase a less resistant band or you can adjust the resistance of your current band. The closer to the ends of the bands you place your hands, the less the resistance. If you are using a looped band, make the loop larger for less resistance.)

If you are able to easily complete 8 to 12 repetitions of an exercise, increase the weight or shorten the length of the band the next time. If you cannot successfully complete 8 to 12 repetitions of an exercise, drop back to a lighter weight or lengthen the band. The ideal weight or length of elastic band is one that makes you feel that the last repetition of an exercise is really all you can do. Remember, no matter the weight or the resistance of the band, 8 to 12 repetitions is a *suggested* goal. If you are only able to complete 1 or 2 reps with a lighter weight or longer band, then that is where you start.

Tips for Using Weights

- It is better to start with too little weight than too much. Too much weight can make you sore, which may discourage you or prevent you from exercising for days.

- Begin each exercise with as many repetitions as you can safely complete. If you can do only three repetitions, then begin there and gradually build to 12, or even 2 sets of 12.

- If you do not have a complete set of weights, select 2 different weights (for example, 2 pounds and 5 pounds) to start. As your strength grows, you can acquire a wider range.

- If your muscles are weak, add just 1 repetition each time you perform an exercise. Eventually, you'll be able to increase the weight as well as the number of repetitions.

- Exercise with weights 2 to 3 times a week on alternate days. Your muscles need a day to rest and rebuild.

Key Points for Strengthening Exercises

- Warm up for approximately 5 minutes before lifting weights. An easy walk or jog while swinging your arms will prepare you for a safe and productive session.

- Complete the entire range of motion for each exercise, being very careful to move slowly and carefully. Do not snap your limbs back to the starting position.

- Perform all movements smoothly. Jerky motion usually indicates that a weight is too heavy.

- Breathing is important. Breathe out as you lift the weights and breathe in as you return to the starting position.

- When an exercise calls for a straight arm or leg position, keep your elbows or knees soft. Do not lock your joints.

- Keep your wrists in a neutral or straight position in most exercises.

- Alternate body parts when you exercise. Start with an arm exercise, followed by 1 for legs, then 1 for neck/trunk. This way you avoid fatiguing one particular body part during your routine. If you decide to do all leg or all arm exercises in a row, then alternate opposing muscle groups. For example, do elbow bends (flexion) followed by elbow straightening (extension).

- Mix isotonic, isometric, and eccentric muscle contractions to help avoid soreness and get the most out of each exercise session. For example, mix the Plank Exercise (Neck and Trunk exercise 8), which is isometric, with Trunk and Hip Bridging (Neck and Trunk exercise 5), which features both eccentric and isotonic contractions.

■ Most strength exercises in this book may be performed using weights or with a Thera-band®. Either method will help you to increase your strength. Bands are great for traveling because they are lightweight and can be used almost anywhere.

Wendy's Prescription for Strength

Wendy's weak areas were her abdominals and back extensors. She decided to do all the exercises in the Neck and Trunk section.

James's Prescription for Strength

James could only extend his back 1 inch during the back extension strength test, and his shoulder blades did not clear the floor in the abdominal strength test. It took him 25 seconds to do the Hip and Knee Strength: Extension, longer than it should have for someone his age. His ankle and toes strength tests also revealed weakness; he could only do 3 toe raises and 2 heel raises. His strengthening program consisted of Neck and Trunk exercises 2, 3, 4, 5, 6, 7, and 8; and Leg exercises 1, 5, 7, and 8. James looks forward to improving his strength to the point at which he only has to perform 2 or 3 exercises.

PRESCRIPTION FOR STRENGTH

Date: _____

Elbow Strength: Flexion
Distance on right: _____
Distance on left: _____
Exercise(s) needed: _____

Elbow Strength: Extension
Distance on right: _____
Distance on left: _____
Exercise(s) needed: _____

Shoulder Strength: Flexion
Distance on right: _____
Distance on left: _____
Exercise(s) needed: _____

Shoulder Strength: Abduction
Distance on right: _____
Distance on left: _____
Exercise(s) needed: _____

Shoulder Strength: Extension
Distance on right: _____
Distance on left: _____
Exercise(s) needed: _____

Hip and Knee Strength: Extension
Time: _____
Exercise(s) needed: _____

Hip Strength: Abduction
Distance on right: _____
Distance on left: _____
Exercise(s) needed: _____

Hip Strength: Flexion
Distance on right: _____
Distance on left: _____
Exercise(s) needed: _____

Knee Strength: Flexion
Distance on right: _____
Distance on left: _____
Exercise(s) needed: _____

Ankle and Toe Strength: Flexion 1
Number on right: _____
Number on left: _____
Exercise(s) needed: _____

Ankle and Toe Strength: Flexion 2
Number on right: _____
Number on left: _____
Exercise(s) needed: _____

Ankle and Toe Strength: Extension
Number on right: _____
Number on left: _____
Exercise(s) needed: _____

Back Strength: Extension
Distance: _____
Exercise(s) needed: _____

Abdominal Strength: Flexion
Distance: _____
Exercise(s) needed: _____

(Make a copy for your personal use)

WHAT IS THE BEST SPEED TO LIFT WEIGHTS ?

This is a controversial question. The information presented in this chapter is based on many studies; however, different views are still evolving. One study published in the *Journal of Sports Medicine and Fitness* showed a 50 percent increase in strength when using the following protocol for strength training developed by Wayne Westcott, an exercise physiologist:

- Do 4 to 6 repetitions per set.
- Take 14 seconds for each repetition: 10 to lift and 4 to lower.
- Each exercise is done using the heaviest weight you can lift slowly 4 to 6 times. If you complete an exercise and feel that you could lift the weight more times, then increase the weight the next time you do the exercise.

BE CREATIVE

How many pennies equal a pound?

Answer: 150.

If you don't have any weights, collect pennies in a plastic bag or sock and use that to get started with your strength-training program.

Other items found around the home that you can use include cans of soup, bags of rice or beans, a plastic tennis ball container filled with sand, plastic bottles—anything that you can comfortably and safely grip in your hands.

8 GREAT EXERCISES FOR ARMS

#1 ■ Overhead Lifts

Why this exercise? This exercise strengthens the muscles that enable you to lift your arms over your head. It will improve your ability to lift objects overhead and will develop and define your muscles from your shoulder to the middle of your upper arm.

1. Sit in a supportive, armless chair, keeping your stomach and chin tucked in so that your back and neck are well aligned. Holding the weights, bend your elbows and raise your arms, moving them out to the side and just above your shoulders. Keep your palms facing forward and your elbows pointing down and out. Breathe in (photo 1).

2. As you breathe out, straighten your arms and slowly lift the weights overhead (photo 2).

3. Slowly lower the weights to the starting position as you breathe in.

4. Do 1 to 2 sets of 8 to 12 repetitions of this exercise.

5. Perform this exercise 3 times a week, every other day.

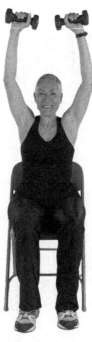
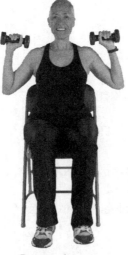

PHOTO 1   PHOTO 2

To perform this exercise with a Thera-band®:

1. Sit in a supportive, armless chair, keeping your stomach and chin tucked in so that your back and neck are well aligned. Place the band under the seat of the chair. Hold the ends of the band in your hands. Bend your elbows and raise your arms, moving them out to the side and just above your shoulders. Keep your palms facing forward and your elbows pointing down and out. Breathe in (photo 3).

2. As you breathe out, straighten your arms and slowly raise your arms overhead (photo 4).

3. Bend your elbows and slowly lower your arms to the starting position as you breathe in.

4. If this is too easy, shorten the band. If this is too hard, do 1 arm at a time. Place 1 hand in your lap and perform the exercise with the other.

5. Do 1 to 2 sets of 8 to 12 repetitions of this exercise.

6. Perform this exercise 3 times a week, every other day.

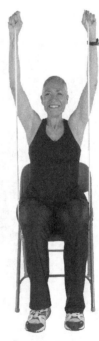

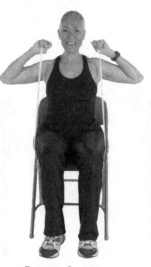

PHOTO 3   PHOTO 4

#2 ■ Upright Rows

Why this exercise? Like Overhead Lifts, this exercise strengthens the muscles that enable you to lift your arms. It will improve your posture and will develop and define your upper back, chest, and shoulder muscles.

1. Sit in a supportive, armless chair, keeping your stomach and chin tucked in so that your back and neck are well aligned. Bend your elbows and hold the weights over your thighs with your palms facing down. Breathe in (photo 1).

2. As you breathe out, slowly lift the weights until they are under your chin. Keep your elbows bent and your arms out to the side and a little higher than your hands (photo 2).

3. Slowly lower the weights to the starting position as you breathe in.

4. Do 1 to 2 sets of 8 to 12 repetitions of this exercise.

5. Perform this exercise 3 times a week, every other day.

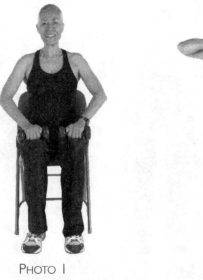
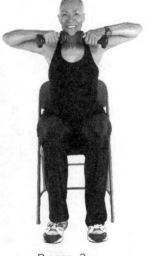

PHOTO 1   PHOTO 2

To perform this exercise with a Thera-band®:

1. Stand up and place the band under your feet. Keep your stomach and chin tucked in so that your back and neck are well aligned. Hold the ends of the band in your hands. Breathe in (photo 3).

2. As you breathe out, slowly raise your arms until your hands are under your chin. Keep your elbows bent and your arms out to the side and a little higher than your hands (photo 4).

3. Slowly lower your arms to the starting position as you breathe in.

4. If this is too easy, shorten the band. If this is too hard, do 1 arm at a time. Place 1 hand in front of your lower abdomen and perform the exercise with the other.

5. You may also do this exercise sitting in a supportive, armless chair. Place the band under the seat of the chair and hold the ends of the band in your hands.

6. Do 1 to 2 sets of 8 to 12 repetitions of this exercise.

7. Perform this exercise 3 times a week, every other day.

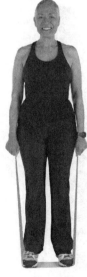
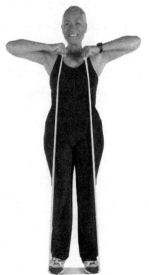

PHOTO 3   PHOTO 4

#3 ■ Shrugs

Why this exercise? This exercise strengthens the muscles that enable you to straighten your upper back and neck. It will improve your ability to lift objects, will keep your head aligned and your neck stable, and will develop and define your neck and upper shoulder muscles. In addition, it will teach you to relax tight neck and shoulder muscles.

1. Sit in a supportive armless chair, keeping your stomach and chin tucked in so that your back and neck are well aligned. Hold the weights at your sides with your arms straight and your palms facing your sides. Breathe in (photo 1).

2. As you breathe out, slowly raise your shoulders toward your ears (photo 2).

3. Slowly lower your shoulders to the starting position and relax your muscles as you breathe in.

4. Do 1 to 2 sets of 8 to 12 repetitions of this exercise.

5. Perform this exercise 3 times a week, every other day.

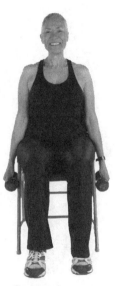
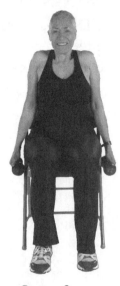

PHOTO 1   PHOTO 2

To perform this exercise with a Thera-band®:

1. Stand up and place the band under your feet. Keep your stomach and chin tucked in so that your back and neck are well aligned. Hold the ends of the band in your hands. Breathe in (photo 3).

2. As you breathe out, slowly raise your shoulders toward your ears (photo 4).

3. Slowly lower your shoulders to the starting position and relax your muscles as you breathe in.

4. If this is too easy, shorten the band. If this is too hard, do 1 arm at a time. Place the band under both of your feet.

5. You may also do this exercise sitting in a supportive, armless chair. Place the band under the seat of the chair and hold the ends of the band in your hands.

6. Do 1 to 2 sets of 8 to 12 repetitions of this exercise.

7. Perform this exercise 3 times a week, every other day.

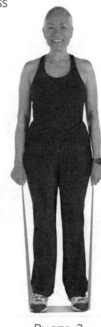

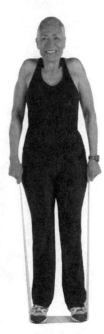

PHOTO 3   PHOTO 4

#4 ■ Shoulder Flexions

Why this exercise? This exercise strengthens the muscles that enable you to lift your arms to the front. It will improve your ability to carry objects and will develop and define the muscles in the front of your shoulders. **Note:** If you have difficulty raising both arms simultaneously, you may do this exercise 1 arm at a time.

1. Sit in a supportive, armless chair, keeping your stomach and chin tucked in so that your back and neck are well aligned. Hold the weights at your sides with your arms straight, your palms facing the chair, and your thumbs facing forward. Breathe in (photo 1).

2. As you breathe out, slowly lift the weights up and to the front, until they are at shoulder height. Keep your elbows soft or slightly bent (photo 2).

3. Slowly lower the weights to the starting position as you breathe in.

4. Do 1 to 2 sets of 8 to 12 repetitions of this exercise.

5. Perform this exercise 3 times a week, every other day.

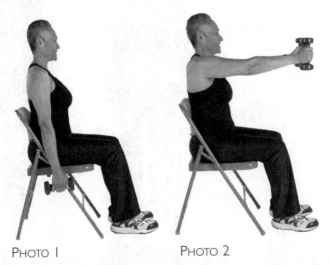

PHOTO 1   PHOTO 2

To perform this exercise with a Thera-band®:

1. Stand up and place the band under your feet. Keep your stomach and chin tucked in so that your back and neck are well aligned. Hold the ends of the band in your hands. Breathe in (photo 3).

2. As you breathe out, slowly raise your arms up and to the front, until they are at shoulder height. Keep your elbows soft or slightly bent (photo 4).

3. Slowly lower your arms to the starting position as you breathe in.

4. If this is too easy, shorten the band. If this is too hard, do 1 arm at a time. Place 1 hand in front of your lower abdomen and perform the exercise with the other.

5. You may also do this exercise sitting in a supportive, armless chair. Place the band under the seat of the chair and hold the ends of the band in your hands.

6. Do 1 to 2 sets of 8 to 12 repetitions of this exercise.

7. Perform this exercise 3 times a week, every other day.

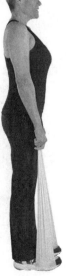
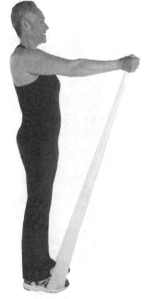

PHOTO 3   PHOTO 4

#5 ■ Shoulder Abductions

Why this exercise? This exercise strengthens the muscles that enable you to lift your arms to the side. It will improve your ability to carry objects and will develop and define the muscles on the sides of your shoulders.

1. Sit in a supportive, armless chair, keeping your stomach and chin tucked in so that your back and neck are well aligned. Hold the weights at your sides with your arms straight, your palms facing the chair, and your thumbs facing forward. Breathe in (photo 1).

2. As you breathe out, raise your arms out to the side until they are at shoulder height. Keep your elbows soft or slightly bent (photo 2).

3. Slowly lower the weights to the starting position as you breathe in.

4. Do 1 to 2 sets of 8 to 12 repetitions of this exercise.

5. Perform this exercise 3 times a week, every other day.

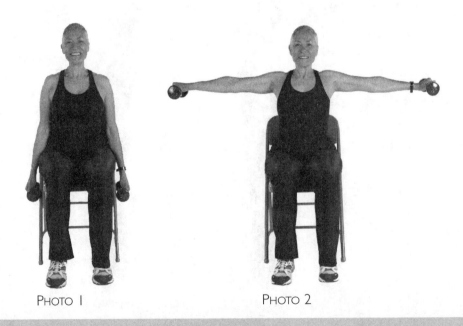

PHOTO 1   PHOTO 2

To perform this exercise with a Thera-band®:

1. Stand up and place the band under your feet. Keep your stomach and chin tucked in so that your back and neck are well aligned. Hold the ends of the band in your hands. Breathe in (photo 3).

2. As you breathe out, raise your arms out to the sides until they are at shoulder height. Keep your elbows soft or slightly bent (photo 4).

3. Slowly lower your arms to the starting position as you breathe in.

4. If this is too easy, shorten the band. If this is too hard, do 1 arm at a time. Place 1 hand in front of your lower abdomen and perform the exercise with the other.

5. You may also do this exercise sitting in a supportive, armless chair. Place the band under the seat of the chair and hold the ends of the band in your hands.

6. Do 1 to 2 sets of 8 to 12 repetitions of this exercise.

7. Perform this exercise 3 times a week, every other day.

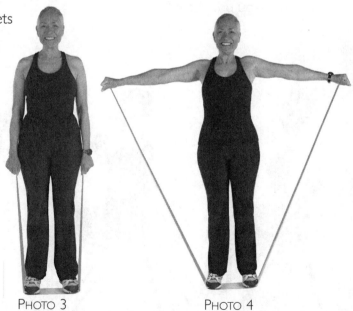

PHOTO 3   PHOTO 4

#6 ■ Elbow Flexions

Why this exercise? This exercise strengthens the muscles that enable you to bend your elbow. These muscles may be relatively strong because you use them frequently when you carry things like groceries, books, or your briefcase. However, if your elbow flexors are weak, this exercise will make it much easier for you. It will help develop and define the muscles in the front of your upper arms. The exercise includes 3 different hand positions.

1. Sit in a supportive, armless chair, keeping your stomach and chin tucked in so that your back and neck are well aligned. Hold the weights at your side with your arms straight. Your palms should face forward (inset 1). Breathe in (photo 1).

2. As you breathe out, bend your elbows and slowly lift the weights toward your shoulders (photo 2).

3. Straighten your elbows and slowly lower the weights to the starting position as you breathe in.

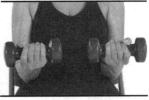

INSET 1

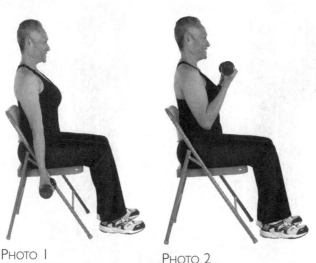

PHOTO 1   PHOTO 2

4. Breathe out and turn your hands so that your thumbs face up (inset 2). Breathe in.

5. As you breathe out, bend your elbows and slowly lift the weights toward your shoulders.

6. Straighten your elbows and slowly lower the weights to the starting position as you breathe in.

7. Breathe out and turn your hands so that your palms face down (inset 3). Breathe in.

8. As you breathe out, bend your elbows and slowly lift the weights toward your shoulders.

9. Straighten your elbows and slowly lower the weights to the starting position as you breathe in.

10. Do 1 to 2 sets of 8 to 12 repetitions of this exercise.

11. Perform this exercise 3 times a week, every other day.

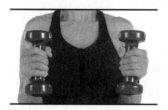

INSET 2

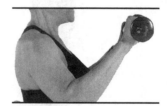

INSET 3

To perform this exercise with a Thera-band®:

1. Stand up and place the band under your feet. Keep your stomach and chin tucked in so that your back and neck are well aligned. Hold the ends of the band in your hands with your thumbs facing forward. Breathe in (photo 3).

2. As you breathe out, bend your elbows and slowly raise your hands toward your shoulders (photo 4).

3. Straighten your elbows and slowly lower your hands to the starting position as you breathe in.

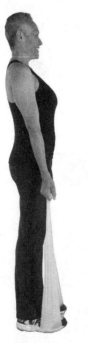 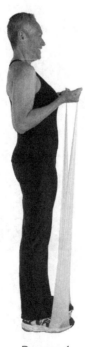

4. Breathe out and turn your hands so that your thumbs face up. Breathe in.

5. As you breathe out, bend your elbows and slowly raise your hands toward your shoulders.

6. Straighten your elbows and slowly lower your hands to the starting position as you breathe in.

7. Breathe in and turn your hand so that your palms face down. Breathe in.

PHOTO 3   PHOTO 4

8. As you breathe out, bend your elbows and slowly raise your hands toward your shoulders.

9. Straighten your elbows and slowly lower your hands to the starting position as you breathe in.

10. If this is too easy, shorten the band. If this is too hard, do 1 arm at a time. Place 1 hand in front of your lower abdomen and perform the exercise with the other.

11. You may also do this exercise sitting in a supportive, armless chair. Place the band under the seat of the chair and hold the ends of the band in your hands.

12. Do 1 to 2 sets of 8 to 12 repetitions of this exercise.

13. Perform this exercise 3 times a week, every other day.

#7 ■ Elbow Extensions

Why this exercise? This exercise strengthens the muscles that enable you to straighten your elbow. It will improve your ability to push with your arms, such as when you push open a door or push yourself up from a chair. It will develop and define the muscles in the back of your upper arm.

1. Sit in a supportive, armless chair, keeping your stomach and chin tucked in so that your back and neck are well aligned. Hold the weights behind your head with your elbows bent, close to your head, and pointed toward the ceiling. Keep your upper arms in line with your ears. Breathe in (photo 1).

2. As you breathe out, slowly straighten your elbows and lift the weights above your head (photo 2).

3. Slowly bend your elbows and lower the weights to the starting position as you breathe in.

4. Do 1 to 2 sets of 8 to 12 repetitions of this exercise.

5. Perform this exercise 3 times a week, every other day.

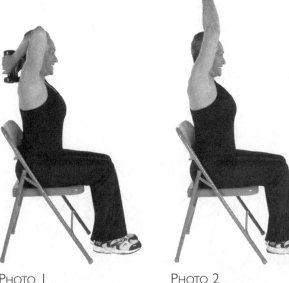

PHOTO 1   PHOTO 2

Note: if you have difficulty extending both elbows simultaneously, you may do this exercise 1 arm at a time.

1. Sit in a supportive, armless chair, keeping your stomach and chin tucked in so that your back and neck are well aligned. Hold the weight in your right hand behind your head with your elbow bent, close to your head, and pointed toward the ceiling. Keep your upper arm in line with your ear. Hold your right elbow with your left hand for support. Breathe in (photo 3).

2. As you breathe out, slowly straighten your elbow and lift the weight above your head. Continue to support your right elbow with your left hand (photo 4).

3. Slowly bend your elbow and lower the weight to the starting position as you breathe in.

4. Repeat the exercise with your left arm.

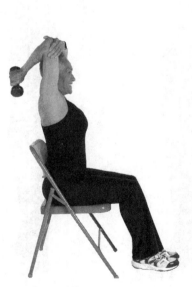
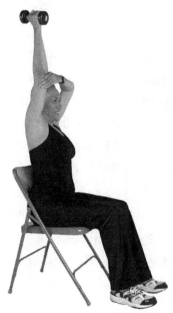

PHOTO 3   PHOTO 4

To perform this exercise with a Thera-band®:

1. Stand up and wrap the band behind your back and under your arms. Hold the ends of the band in your hands. Keep your stomach and chin tucked in so that your back and neck are well aligned. Bend your elbows. Raise your arms over your head, keeping your elbows close to your head and pointed toward the ceiling. Keep your upper arms in line with your ears. Breathe in (photo 5).

2. As you breathe out, slowly straighten your elbows and lift your hands over your head (photo 6).

3. Slowly bend your elbows and return to the starting position as you breathe in.

4. If this is too easy, shorten the band. If this is too hard, do 1 arm at a time. Keep 1 arm bent , the hand at your shoulder and the elbow pointing down; perform the exercise with your other arm.

5. You may also do this exercise sitting in a supportive, armless chair. Place the band under the seat of the chair and hold the ends of the band in your hands.

6. Do 1 to 2 sets of 8 to 12 repetitions of this exercise.

7. Perform this exercise 3 times a week, every other day.

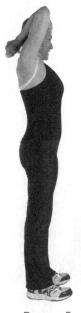

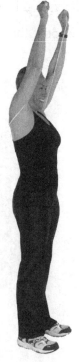

Photo 5　　　　　　　　Photo 6

#8 ■ Shoulder Extensions

Why this exercise? This exercise strengthens the muscles that enable you to raise your arms to the back. It will improve your ability to lift objects more easily and develop and define the muscles in the back of your shoulders.

1. Stand up. Put your left foot in front of your right foot and slightly bend your knees. Keep your feet parallel. Bend over and rest your left forearm on your left thigh. Hold the weight in your right arm and let your right arm hang down. Breathe in (photo 1). Keep your back straight and your neck aligned with your spine. Don't lift your head as you perform this exercise (inset).

2. As you breathe out, raise your right arm up toward the ceiling (photo 2).

3. Slowly lower your arm as you straighten your elbow, and return to the starting position as you breathe in.

4. Repeat the exercise with your left arm.

5. Do 1 to 2 sets of 8 to 12 repetitions of this exercise on each side.

6. Perform this exercise 3 times a week, every other day.

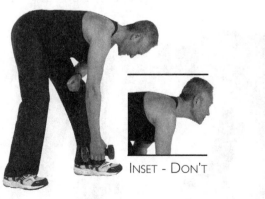

INSET - DON'T

PHOTO 1

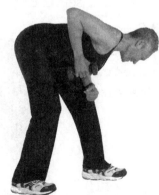

PHOTO 2

To perform this exercise with a Thera-band®:

1. Stand up. Put your left foot in front of your right foot and slightly bend your knees. Keep your feet parallel. Place the middle of the band under your right foot. Hold both ends of the band in your right hand. Bend over, keeping your right arm by your side with the elbow bent. Rest your left forearm against your left thigh. Breathe in (photo 3). Keep your back straight and your neck aligned with your spine. Don't lift your head as you perform this exercise.

2. As you breathe out, raise your right elbow toward the ceiling (photo 4).

3. Slowly lower your arm, straighten your elbow, and return to the starting position as you breathe in.

4. Repeat the exercise with your left arm.

5. If this is too easy, shorten the band. If this is too hard, hold the band closer to the ends so that it is longer.

6. You may also do this exercise sitting in a supportive, armless chair. Place the band under the seat of the chair and hold the ends in your hands.

7. Do 1 to 2 sets of 8 to 12 repetitions of this exercise on each side.

8. Perform this exercise 3 times a week, every other day.

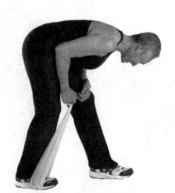
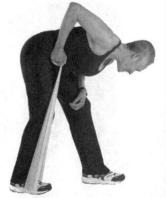

PHOTO 3   PHOTO 4

8 GREAT EXERCISES FOR LEGS

#1 Hip Extensions on All Fours

#2 Hip Flexions

#3 Hip Abductions

#4 Hip Adductions

#5 Wall Slides

#6 Knee Flexions

#7 Toe Rises

#8 Toes Up

#1 ■ Hip Extensions on All Fours

Why this exercise? This exercise strengthens the muscles that help you walk efficiently, rise from a chair quickly, and climb stairs easily. It will counteract the negative effects of sitting for long periods and will develop and define the muscles in your buttocks and the backs of your legs. You may perform this exercise with or without cuff weights around your ankles.

1. Get on your hands and knees. Tighten your stomach and tuck in your chin so that your back is straight. Breathe in (photo 1).

2. As you breathe out, slowly straighten and raise your right leg, keeping your weight on your left knee (photo 2). Keep your back straight and do not lean forward or back. Do not raise your right leg above the line of your back and neck.

3. Slowly lower your leg to the starting position as you breathe in.

4. Repeat the exercise with your left leg.

5. Do 1 to 2 sets of 8 to 12 repetitions of this exercise on each side.

6. Perform this exercise 3 times a week, every other day.

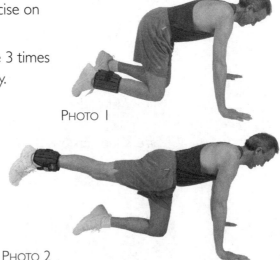

PHOTO 1

PHOTO 2

To perform this exercise with a Thera-band®:

1. Tie the ends of the band together tightly to make a loop. Get on your hands and knees. Put the loop around your legs so that you are kneeling on it with your left leg and it is behind your right knee. Tighten your stomach and tuck in your chin so that your back is straight. Breathe in.

2. As you breathe out, slowly straighten and raise your right leg, keeping your weight on your left knee (photo 3). Keep your back straight and do not lean forward or back. Do not raise your right leg above the line of your back and neck.

3. Slowly lower your leg to the starting position as you breathe in.

4. Repeat the exercise with your left leg.

5. If this is too easy, shorten the band by making a smaller loop. If this is too hard, lengthen the band by making a larger loop.

6. Do 1 to 2 sets of 8 to 12 repetitions of this exercise on each side.

7. Perform this exercise 3 times a week, every other day.

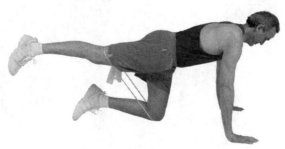

Photo 3

#2 ■ Hip Flexions

Why this exercise? This exercise strengthens the muscles that help you lift your leg when you ascend steps or curbs. It will develop and define the muscles in the front of your hip. If you are having difficulty lifting your leg high enough to get on a bus or into your car or you are having difficulty when you start to walk, you should work on strengthening these muscles. You may perform this exercise with or without cuff weights around your ankles.

1. Stand. If you need help balancing, lightly place 1 or 2 fingers on the back of a sturdy chair or a counter. Tighten your stomach and tuck in your chin so that your back is straight. Breathe in (photo 1).

2. As you breathe out, slowly bend your right knee and raise your right leg until your thigh is parallel to the floor (photo 2). Keep your back straight and do not bend forward or lean back.

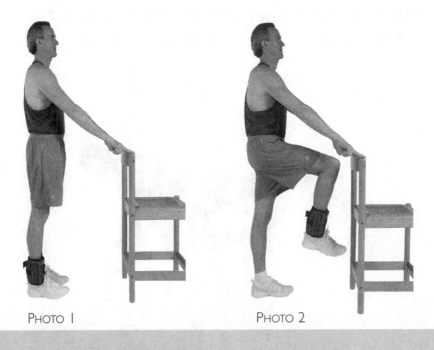

PHOTO 1   PHOTO 2

3. Slowly lower your leg to the starting position as you breathe in.

4. Repeat the exercise with your left leg.

5. Do 1 to 2 sets of 8 to 12 repetitions of this exercise on each side.

6. Perform this exercise 3 times a week, every other day.

To perform this exercise with a Thera-band®:

1. Tie the ends of the band together tightly to make a loop. Stand on the loop; raise your right foot so that the band is under your left foot and on top of your right foot. Tighten your stomach and tuck in your chin so that your back is straight. Breathe in.

2. As you breathe out, slowly bend your right knee and raise your right leg until your thigh is parallel to the floor (photo 3). Keep your back straight and do not bend forward or lean back.

3. Slowly lower your leg to the starting position as you breathe in.

4. Repeat the exercise with your left leg.

5. If this is too easy, shorten the band by making a smaller loop. If this is too hard, lengthen the band by making a larger loop.

6. Do 1 to 2 sets of 8 to 12 repetitions of this exercise on each side.

7. Perform this exercise 3 times a week, every other day.

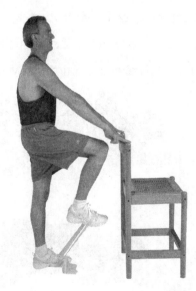

PHOTO 3

#3 ■ Hip Abductions

Why this exercise? This exercise strengthens the muscles that help keep your pelvis level while you walk, enabling you to hold your body in a more stable position. It will develop and define the muscles in your outer hip and buttocks, which can be weakened by many things, including minor ankle sprains (even early in life), knee cartilage problems, and hip replacements. You may perform this exercise with or without cuff weights around your ankles.

1. Lie on the floor on your right side. Keep your back against a wall so that you are correctly aligned. Put a pillow under your head. Tighten your stomach and tuck in your chin so that your back is straight. Bend your right knee and bring your right leg toward your chest, keeping your left leg straight. Breathe in (photo 1).

2. As you breathe out, slowly raise your left leg 6 to 8 inches (photo 2).

3. Slowly lower your left leg to the starting position as you breathe in.

4. Repeat the exercise with your right leg.

5. Do 1 to 2 sets of 8 to 12 repetitions of this exercise on each side.

6. Perform this exercise 3 times a week, every other day.

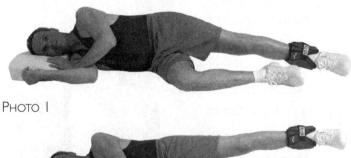

PHOTO 1

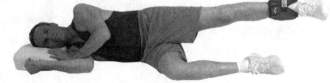

PHOTO 2

To perform this exercise with a Thera-band®:

1. Tie the ends of the band together tightly to make a loop. Lie on the floor on your right side. Put a pillow under your head. Tighten your stomach and tuck in your chin so that your back is straight. Pull the loop up around your thighs, just above your knees. Bend your right knee and bring your right leg toward your chest, keeping your left leg straight. Breathe in.

2. As you breathe out, slowly raise your left leg 6 to 8 inches (photo 3).

3. Slowly lower your left leg to the starting position as you breathe in.

4. Repeat the exercise with your right leg.

5. If this is too easy, shorten the band by making a smaller loop. If this is too hard, lengthen the band by making a larger loop.

6. Do 1 to 2 sets of 8 to 12 repetitions of this exercise on each side.

7. Perform this exercise 3 times a week, every other day.

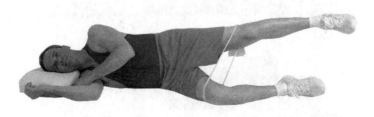

PHOTO 3

#4 ■ Hip Adductions

Why this exercise? This exercise strengthens the muscles you use to cross
your legs and to keep them relatively close together while walking, maintaining
balance and symmetry. It will also make you more stable when you stand and
walk. Though these muscles are rarely weak, they should be exercised to keep
your body balanced. This exercise will develop and define the muscles in your
inner thigh and groin areas. You may perform it with or without cuff weights
around your ankles.

1. Lie on the floor on your right side. Put a pillow under your head.
Tighten your stomach and tuck in your chin so that your back is
straight. Bend your left leg and rest the foot in front of your right
knee. Breathe in (photo 1).

2. Keeping your right leg straight, slowly raise it about 4 inches as you
breathe out (photo 2).

3. Slowly lower your right leg to the starting position as you breathe in.

4. Repeat the exercise with your left leg.

5. Do 1 to 2 sets of 8 to 12 repetitions of this exercise on each side.

6. Perform this exercise 3 times a week, every other day.

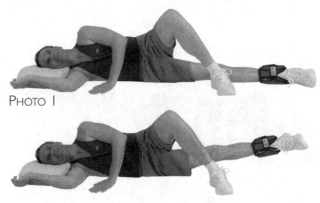

PHOTO 1

PHOTO 2

To perform this exercise with a Thera-band®:

1. Tie the ends of the band together tightly to make a loop. Lie on the floor on your right side. Put a pillow under your head. Tighten your stomach and tuck in your chin so that your back is straight. Place the loop under your left foot and around your right thigh just above your knee. Bend your left leg and rest the foot in front of your right knee. Breathe in.

2. Keeping your right leg straight, slowly raise it about 4 inches as you breathe out (photo 3).

3. Slowly lower your right leg to the starting position as you breathe in.

4. Repeat the exercise with your left leg.

5. If this is too easy, shorten the band by making a smaller loop. If this is too hard, lengthen the band by making a larger loop.

6. Do 1 to 2 sets of 8 to 12 repetitions of this exercise on each side.

7. Perform this exercise 3 times a week, every other day.

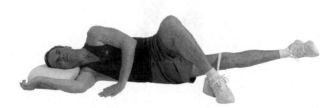

Photo 3

#5 ■ Wall Slides

Why this exercise? Like Hip Extensions, this exercise strengthens the muscles that help you walk efficiently, rise from a chair quickly, and climb stairs easily. It will develop and define the muscles of your buttocks and the fronts of your thighs. Wall Slides are very effective and efficient—which is helpful when you are pressed for time. You may perform this exercise with or without hand weights; if you use weights, you can keep your hands at your sides or place the weights on top of your shoulders.

1. Stand with your arms at your side and your feet parallel and approximately shoulder-width apart, at least 18 to 24 inches away from a wall. Tighten your stomach and tuck in your chin so that your back is straight. Breathe in (photo 1).

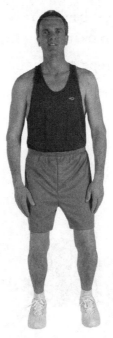

PHOTO 1

2. As you breathe out, slowly bend your knees keeping your back against the wall. Slide your torso down the wall until you are in a sitting position with your knees behind or just over your ankles (photo 2). As you hold this position, be sure to breathe in and out steadily. Count out loud to assure that you are doing so.

3. Slowly straighten your knees, slide back up the wall, and return to the starting position as you breathe in.

4. Perform this exercise 3 times a week, every other day.

Note: To increase the impact of this exercise, stay in the sitting position for increasing periods of time. Begin with 10 seconds, gradually building to 60. Once you are comfortable holding the position for 60 seconds, you may further enhance this exercise's benefits as follows: while holding the position, rise onto your toes, then lower your heels and lift your toes off the floor.

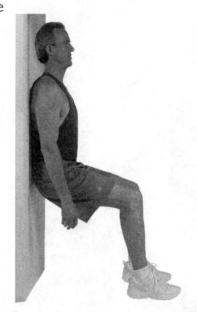

PHOTO 2

#6 ■ Knee Flexions

Why this exercise? This exercise strengthens the muscles that help you bend your knees and control their motion while you walk. The knee flexors (especially the hamstrings) are essential for walking. This exercise will develop and define the muscles in the back of your thighs. You may perform this exercise with or without cuff weights around your ankles.

1. Stand. If you need help balancing, lightly place 1 or 2 fingers on the back of a sturdy chair or a counter. Tighten your stomach and tuck in your chin so that your back is straight. Breathe in (photo 1).

2. As you breathe out, slowly bend your right knee, raising your right calf behind you. Keep your thighs parallel (photo 2).

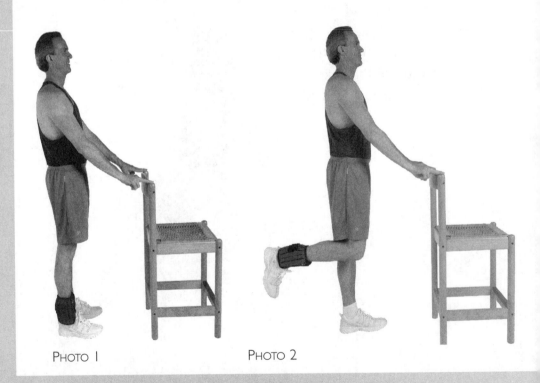

PHOTO 1   PHOTO 2

3. Slowly lower your leg to the starting position as you breathe in.

4. Repeat this exercise with your left leg.

5. Do 1 to 2 sets of 8 to 12 repetitions of this exercise.

6. Perform this exercise 3 times a week, every other day.

To perform this exercise with a Thera-band®:

1. Tie the ends of the band together tightly to make a loop. Stand. Place the loop under your left foot and behind your right ankle. Tighten your stomach and tuck in your chin so that your back is straight. Breathe in.

2. As you breathe out, slowly bend your right knee, raising your right calf behind you. Keep your thighs parallel (photo 3).

3. Slowly lower your leg to the starting position as you breathe in.

4. Repeat this exercise with your left leg.

5. If this is too easy, shorten the band by making a smaller loop. If this is too hard, lengthen the band by making a larger loop.

6. Do 1 to 2 sets of 8 to 12 repetitions of this exercise on each side.

7. Perform this exercise 3 times a week, every other day.

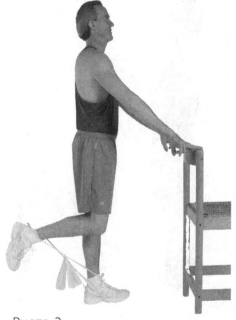

PHOTO 3

#7 ■ Toe Rises

Why this exercise? This exercise strengthens the muscles that help you run, jump, stand, and walk efficiently. These muscles play an important role in many daily activities and help you maintain good balance. This exercise will develop and define the muscles in the backs of your calves. You may perform this exercise with or without cuff weights around your ankles.

1. Stand. If you need help balancing, lightly place 1 or 2 fingers on the back of a sturdy chair or a counter. Tighten your stomach and tuck in your chin so that your back is straight. Breathe in (photo 1).

2. As you breathe out, slowly rise onto your toes (photo 2).

3. Slowly return to the starting position as you breathe in.

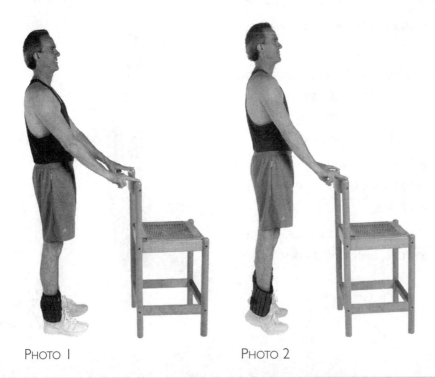

PHOTO 1   PHOTO 2

4. Build up to 50 repetitions of this exercise.

5. Perform this exercise 3 times a week, every other day.

Note: If you have good balance, you can increase the difficulty of this exercise in 3 ways:

■ Don't use the back of the chair or counter for support.

■ Hold weights at your sides or on top of your shoulders.

■ Perform the exercise balancing on 1 leg; keep the other off the floor.

During your day, you have many opportunities to strengthen these muscles:

■ Do Toe Rises while you brush your teeth or wash your face.

■ Walk on your toes several times a day.

#8 ■ Toes Up

Why this exercise? Ever stubbed your toe and then stumbled? This exercise strengthens the muscles that prevent you from dragging your toes when you walk, climb stairs, and step over curbs. These muscles also help you maintain good balance. This exercise will develop and define the muscles in the front of your lower legs. You may perform this exercise with or without cuff weights around your ankles.

1. Stand. If you need help balancing, lightly place 1 or 2 fingers on the back of a sturdy chair or a counter. Tighten your stomach and tuck in your chin so that your back is straight. Breathe in (photo 1).

2. As you breathe out, slowly lift your toes and the balls of your feet off the floor (photo 2).

3. Slowly lower your toes and the balls of your feet back to the starting position as you breathe in.

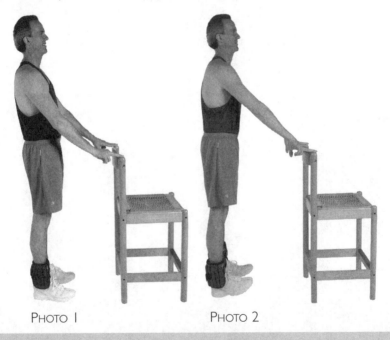

PHOTO 1   PHOTO 2

4. Build up to 50 repetitions of this exercise.

5. Perform this exercise 3 times a week, every other day.

Note: If you have good balance, you can increase the difficulty of this exercise in 3 ways:

■ Don't use the back of a chair or counter for support.

■ Hold weights at your sides or on top of your shoulders.

■ Perform the exercise balanced on one leg; keep the other leg off the floor.

During your day, you have many opportunities to strengthen these muscles:

■ Do Toes Up while you brush your teeth or wash your face.

■ Walk on your heels several times a day.

8 GREAT EXERCISES FOR NECK AND TRUNK

Caution: If you have any neck or lower back pain, consult a physician or physical therapist before doing any of these exercises. **Note:** Several studies have demonstrated that people who do regular exercises similar to Neck Flexions and Extensions and Neck Rotations have less neck pain and fewer neck-related surgeries.

#1 ■ Neck Flexions and Extensions

Why this exercise? This exercise strengthens the muscles that help you hold your head straight and enable you to tuck in your chin, nod, and turn your head. It will develop and define the muscles at the front and back of your neck. This exercise features isometric contractions, as described on page 69. You will exert force but not actually move your head and neck.

1. Lie on your back with your knees bent and your feet flat on the floor. Place one hand at your side and the other against your forehead. Breathe in (photo 1).

2. Push your head against the hand on your forehead, as if you were trying to bring your chin to your chest. Do not allow any movement to occur. Hold this position for 6 to 10 seconds as you breathe out.

3. Put 1 hand behind your head and the other at your side. Relax and breathe in.

4. Push your head back against your hand (photo 2). Do not allow any movement to occur. Hold this position for 6 to 10 seconds as you breathe out.

5. Relax and breathe in.

6. Repeat both movements, building to 10 repetitions.

7. Perform this exercise every day.

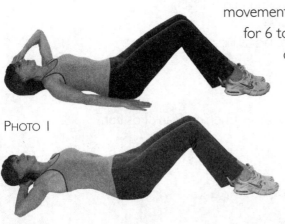

PHOTO 1

PHOTO 2

#2 ■ Neck Rotations

Why this exercise? This exercise strengthens the muscles that enable you to turn your head. It will develop and define the muscles at the front and back of your neck. This exercise features isometric contractions, as described on page 69. You will exert force but not actually move your head and neck.

1. Lie on your back with your knees bent and your feet flat on the floor. Place your right hand on your right temple or cheek and your left hand at your side. Breathe in (photo 1).

2. Push your face against your hand as if you were trying to turn your head to the right. Do not allow any movement to occur. Hold this position for 6 to 10 seconds as you breathe out.

3. Relax and breathe in.

4. Repeat this exercise on your left side.

5. Build to 10 repetitions of this exercise on each side.

6. Perform this exercise every day.

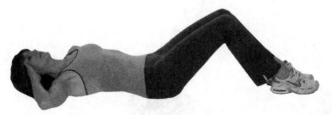

PHOTO 1

#3 ■ Trunk Flexions

Why this exercise? This exercise strengthens the muscles that keep your back well aligned when you stand, as well as the muscles that support your abdomen. It will develop and define your stomach muscles. Though many people want "six-pack abs," they are probably not realistic for most of us. But this exercise will tone your *Rectus abdominus!*

1. Lie on your back with your knees bent and your feet flat on the floor. Put your hands behind your head. Tuck your chin into your chest and keep it there throughout this exercise. Breathe in (photo 1).

2. Using your abdominal muscles, slowly and smoothly raise your head and shoulders. Do not lift your shoulder blades off the floor. Avoid pulling your head up with your hands. Hold this position for 6 to 10 seconds as you breathe out (photo 2).

3. Slowly lower your head and shoulders to the starting position as you breathe in.

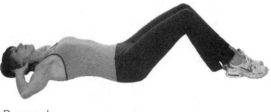

PHOTO 1

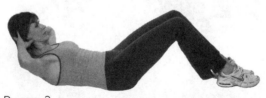

PHOTO 2

4. Do as many repetitions of this exercise as you comfortably can, building to 10.

5. Perform this exercise every day.

Note: You can increase the difficulty of this exercise by varying your leg or arm positions:

■ Straighten and raise your legs and bend your knees approximately 90 degrees. This is called a tabletop position (photos 3 and 4).

■ Straighten and raise your legs and cross your ankles (photo 5).

■ Straighten one or both legs after you raise your head and shoulders (photo 6).

■ Change the position of your arms—cross them on your chest or straighten and raise them overhead, keeping them close to your ears.

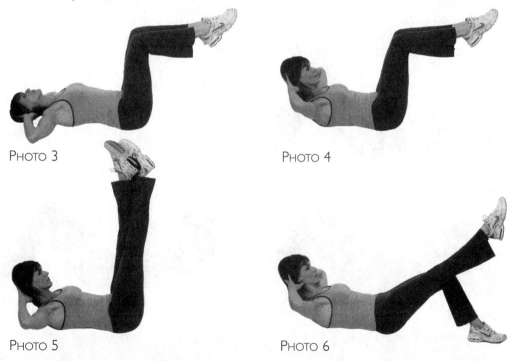

PHOTO 3   PHOTO 4

PHOTO 5   PHOTO 6

#4 ■ Trunk Flexions and Rotations

Why this exercise? This exercise strengthens your internal and external oblique muscles—the ones that enable you to twist and bend your trunk. They help keep your back well aligned while you stand and provide support for your abdomen. Like Trunk Flexions, this exercise will develop and define your stomach muscles.

1. Lie on your back with your knees bent and your feet flat on the floor. Put your hands behind your head. Tuck your chin in to your chest and keep it there throughout this exercise. Breathe in (photo 1).

2. Using your abdominal muscles, slowly and smoothly raise your head and shoulders up and to the right, moving your left elbow toward your right hip (photo 2). Avoid pulling your head up with your hands. Hold this position for 6 to 10 seconds as you breathe out.

3. Slowly lower your head and shoulders to the starting position as you breathe in.

4. Repeat this exercise on the other side (photo 3).

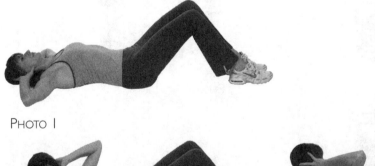

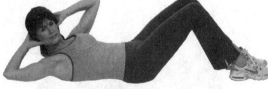

PHOTO 1

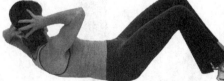

PHOTO 2   PHOTO 3

5. Do as many repetitions of this exercise as you comfortably can, building to 10.

6. Perform this exercise every day.

Note: You can increase the difficulty of this exercise by varying your leg positions:

■ Raise your legs and bend your knees approximately 90 degrees. This is called tabletop position (photos 4 and 5).

■ Straighten and raise your legs and cross your ankles (photo 6).

■ Bicycle your legs: as you reach your right elbow to your left knee, straighten your right leg, then reverse positions.

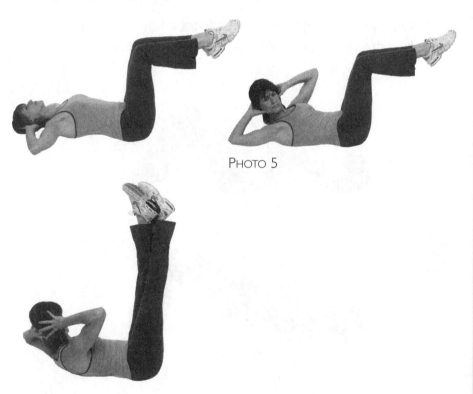

PHOTO 5

PHOTO 6

#5 ■ Trunk and Hip Bridging

Why this exercise? This exercise strengthens the abdominal, back, and buttocks muscles that support your trunk and extend your hips. These are the muscles that help you to rise more easily from a chair and to walk more efficiently. This exercise will develop and define the muscles of your stomach, buttocks, hips, and lower legs.

1. Lie on your back with your knees bent and your feet flat on the floor. Keep your arms at your sides and your palms flat on the floor. Tighten your stomach muscles and tuck in your chin. Breathe in (photo 1).

2. Slowly and smoothly raise your buttocks off the floor, keeping your back straight. Hold this position for 6 to 10 seconds as you breathe out (photo 2).

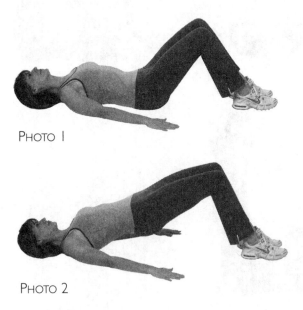

Photo 1

Photo 2

3. Slowly lower your buttocks to the starting position as you breathe in.

4. Build to holding this position for 1 minute.

5. Perform this exercise every day.

Note: As you get stronger, try straightening one leg while you hold the position (photo 3).

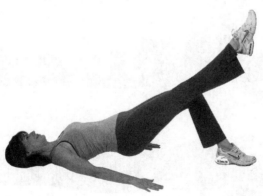

PHOTO 3

#6 ■ Scapula Stabilization

Why this exercise? This exercise strengthens the muscles that help keep your shoulder blades properly aligned and stabilized while you stand. It will help your arms function more efficiently and is indispensable if you play golf or tennis. This exercise will develop and define the muscles in your upper back and between your shoulder blades. If you want good posture and a better toned upper back, you must do this exercise. You may perform it with or without hand weights. These muscles are often not very strong, so start with no weight or very light weights and gradually build up.

1. Lie facedown on the floor with a large pillow under your stomach. Rest your forehead on the floor or on a small, rolled towel. Bend your elbows at a 90-degree angle and place your forearms on the floor. Tighten your stomach muscles and tuck in your chin. Breathe in (photo 1).

2. Keeping your forehead on the floor or the towel, smoothly raise your arms as high as comfortably possible. Hold this position for 6 to 10 seconds as you breathe out (photo 2).

3. Slowly lower your arms to the starting position as you breathe in.

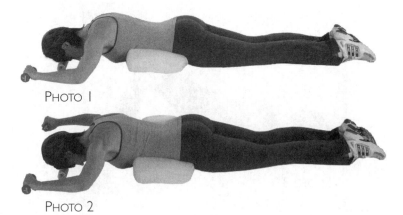

PHOTO 1

PHOTO 2

4. Build to 10 repetitions of this exercise.

5. Perform this exercise every day.

To perform this exercise with a Thera-band®:

1. Lie facedown on the floor with a large pillow under your stomach. Rest your forehead on the floor or on a small, rolled towel. Bend your elbows at a 90-degree angle and place your forearms on the floor.

2. Place the band under your upper abdomen. Hold the ends of the band in your hands. Tighten your stomach muscles and tuck in your chin. Breathe in.

3. Keeping your forehead on the floor or the towel, smoothly raise your arms as high as comfortably possible. Hold this position for 6 to 10 seconds as you breathe out (photo 3).

4. Slowly lower your arms to the starting position as you breathe in.

5. Build to 10 repetitions of this exercise.

6. Perform this exercise every day.

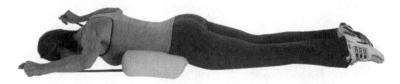

PHOTO 3

#7 ■ Trunk Extensions

Why this exercise? This exercise strengthens the muscles that help to keep your trunk straight while you stand and enable you to move your trunk more quickly and efficiently. It will help relieve the fatigue that can occur when you sit for prolonged periods of time. It will also develop and define your back muscles. **Caution:** If you have back problems, consult your physcial therapist or physician before doing this exercise.

1. Lie facedown on the floor with a large pillow under your stomach. Rest your forehead on the floor or on a small, rolled towel. Stretch your arms out over your head, keeping them close to your ears. Tighten your stomach muscles and tuck in your chin; keep them tight and tucked throughout this exercise. Breathe in (photo 1).

2. At the same time, raise your right arm and your left leg about 1 inch off the floor, keeping them both straight. Smoothly stretch them in opposite directions as far as is comfortable, as if someone were pulling your arm forward and your leg backward (photo 2). Hold this position for 6 to 10 seconds as you breathe out.

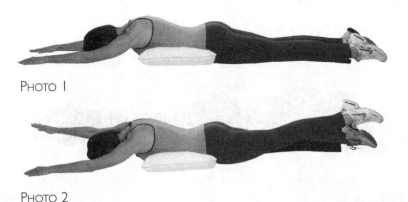

PHOTO 1

PHOTO 2

3. Return your arm and leg to their starting positions as you breathe in.

4. Repeat this exercise, using your left arm and right leg.

5. Build to 10 repetitions of this exercise.

6. Perform this exercise every day.

Note: You may also do this exercise on your hands and knees, but remember that it also requires balance to do it in this position (photo 3).

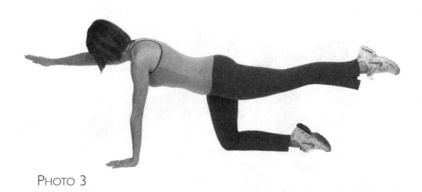

PHOTO 3

#8 ■ Trunk Strengthening: Plank Position

Why this exercise? This exercise strengthens almost all of the muscles of your body. It will develop and define many of the muscles in your neck, trunk, arms, and legs. This is probably the toughest exercise in the book. It's especially effective because it contracts so many of your muscles at the same time. If you are pressed for time and want to get the maximum strengthening benefit from just 1 activity, do this exercise.

1. Get on your hands and knees, keeping your hands aligned under your shoulders. Tighten your stomach and tuck in your chin so that your back is straight. Breathe in (photo 1).

2. Straighten your right leg and move it behind you; do the same with your left leg. Keep your toes curled and your body perfectly

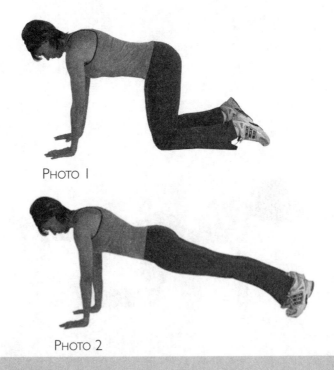

PHOTO 1

PHOTO 2

straight (photo 2). Hold this position for 6 to 10 seconds, being sure to breathe in and out regularly. It may help to count out loud.

3. Breathe out and return to the starting position.

4. Build to holding this position for 1 minute.

5. Perform this exercise every day.

Note: When you start doing this exercise, hold the position for no more than 6 to 10 seconds. To do this exercise properly, you must maintain correct alignment; the longer you hold this position, the harder it gets to do that. As you become stronger, you may hold the position for longer periods of time. We give "Plank Awards" to our clients who can hold the position correctly for 1 minute or longer.

HOW TO CREATE A STRENGTH TRAINING ROUTINE

If you had difficulty with any part of the strength assessment, consider beginning a regular training program. Reassess your performance every 2 months. Once you can easily pass each of the strength tests, you can reduce your program to 1 set of each exercise, performed 2 or 3 times a week. Before beginning a program take special note of these recommendations:

■ Review Tips for Using Weights and Key Points for Strengthening Exercises (pages 86–88).

■ If you cannot successfully complete 8 to 12 repetitions of each exercise, lower the weight for your next session.

■ The first time you try an exercise, see how many repetitions you can perform. If it is only 2 or 3, that's fine—that's where your program starts.

■ If you are able to do 8 to 12 repetitions completely and easily, increase the weight for your next session.

■ When you perform exercises that do not use weights or the Thera-band®, try increasing the repetitions every other session. Reach for a goal of 50 to 100 repetitions.

DAILY TIPS AND ENERGIZING IDEAS

This section includes easy-to-do tasks, modifications to daily activities, and tips to enhance and reinforce the exercises in your strength program. Place little notes to yourself everywhere you tend to look during the day. as reminders to do them every day.

AT HOME AND WORK

■ Do a little more each day. For example, walk up another flight of stairs or lift a few more plates onto a shelf.

■ If you sit for 5 hours or more each day, take a 5-minute walk every 30 to 40 minutes.

■ If you get up from your chair only 6 times a day, increase that to 8, then 10 times a day. Before you stand, push your elbows into the back rest of your chair 3 to 5 times to help straighten your spine. Then shift to the front of the chair and stand up slowly, keeping your body perfectly straight and using only your legs. Stand up and sit down 5 times before getting up to go for your walk.

■ If you exercise 15 minutes each day, increase your time to 30, then to 40 minutes each day.

■ If other people usually get items for you, get them for yourself.

■ Tighten your stomach and tuck in your chin when you prepare meals, dress, shave, put on makeup, or sit.

■ Avoid long, static (isometric) contractions of your muscles. For example, don't keep your hands, elbows, and arms in the same position when you carry groceries. Raise and lower your hands or change the side on which you carry the bag. Also, try to carry a balanced load—things of equal weight in each hand or over both shoulders in a backpack.

■ Take the stairs instead of the elevator whenever you can.

■ When you're standing still, use the time to exercise. For example, if you are in an elevator, do Toe Rises or Toes Up; if you are in the car, tuck in your chin and tighten your stomach muscles while you are stopped at traffic lights.

■ Take your Thera-band® with you when you travel.

■ While you watch TV, push both elbows back into your chair as you tighten your stomach and chin to strengthen your upper back. Squeeze your buttocks together so that you sit taller. Press your toes into the floor.

■ When you sit, do isometric exercises using your hands for resistance. Push your hands against the outsides of your upper legs as you try to force your thighs apart for 6 to 10 seconds. Place your left hand on your right forearm and bend your right elbow while resisting the movement.

IN THE GYM

■ All of the strength exercises may also be done at the gym. Use free and cuff weights or the various exercise machines. Because equipment varies from one place to another, make sure that you receive appropriate instruction before you use each machine.

■ Follow the guidelines for each exercise.

■ Be very aware of proper breathing techniques and good postural alignment.

■ To avoid fatiguing any one set of muscles, vary your routine. Try using a machine for arms, followed by one for legs, followed by one for the trunk. If this is not possible, at least exercise opposing muscle groups (for example, biceps followed by triceps or quadriceps followed by hamstrings).

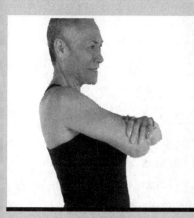

Chapter 4

Balance

USING VISUALIZATION TO INCREASE BALANCE

An impressive study in the journal *Physical Therapy* compared balance in 2 groups of women. As they performed various balance activities, the first group listened to a visualization/relaxation tape, the second to music. The researcher observed huge improvements in balance in the group that listened to the visualization/relaxation tape.

Positive visualization will enhance the balance exercises in this book. For example, while balancing, you could imagine being caressed by a cool, calm breeze, or while standing on 1 leg, you could pretend you are a brightly colored bird or a straight, tall tree. Think back to balance games you played as a child, such as walking along a curb or on the top of a low wall, and incorporate those images into your visualization.

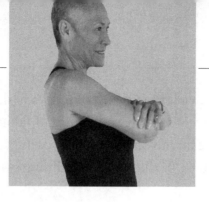

I smoke cigars because at my age
if I don't have something to hold onto, I might fall down.

—GEORGE BURNS

Many of us are looking for balance in our lives. Balance—in both the social and physical sense of the word—is indispensable to healthy living, particularly as people live longer. In the United States, the segment of the population that has experienced the largest growth is composed of people 100 years or older. If we are going to live both long and well, a good sense of balance is essential.

Research shows that one-third of people over the age of 65 falls at least once each year, and these falls can have devastating consequences. But bruises and broken bones are not the only unfortunate results from a loss of balance. People prone to falling must limit their activities; many of them experience unhappiness, anxiety, loss of independence, and even life-threatening complications.

Ruby, a 67-year-old grandmother, greatly feared falling. Many of her friends had fallen and broken bones or ended up using walkers. Because she was so afraid of losing her balance, she was becoming less and less active and now passed up most invitations to go out.

Falls often lead to a vicious cycle: a fall results in decreased activity, which reduces stability, increasing the chance of falling again. Studies show that if you take care of yourself by improving your balance—as well as your posture, strength, flexibility, and endurance—you are much less likely to fall.

PROPER BALANCE

Balance is the ability of your body to maintain equilibrium when you stand, walk, or perform any other daily activity. It is based on input from different body systems and is influenced by many different factors. There are 2 primary types of balance:

Static balance is the ability to maintain a position without moving. It allows you to balance on 1 foot while you pull on your pants, to stand upright for prolonged periods of time, or to reach away from your body in any direction without falling. Many daily tasks require steadiness while reaching forward, backward, to the right, and to the left.

Moving balance is the ability to maintain balanced posture while moving. It allows you to maintain an upright position while you walk or climb curbs, stairs, ramps, or a ladder.

BALANCE CHANGES

Many age-related changes may affect balance. Vision problems, including degeneration of the nerves between the brain and eyes, atrophy of eye muscles, cataracts, glaucoma, macular degeneration, and loss of eye lens elasticity, can lead to falls. Hearing problems, resulting from the degeneration of the nerves between the brain and ears, may also decrease balance.

Changes in your brain, including the thickening of its lining, a reduction in its total size, and an increase in fat in its pathways, may result in decreased perception. These changes, particularly in the lower portions of the brain, may lead to problems in coordination and timing of movements.

Reduction in muscle strength may force you to work harder to obtain the same results that you used to achieve with less work. Your reaction time may be delayed, which increases your chance of a fall. Decreased proprioception—your awareness of your postural alignment, movement, and position change—may also affect your sense of balance.

More than the other domains, balance problems can have devastating results, including falls that result in injuries, hospitalizations, and surgeries. With regular training, however, muscles, joint receptors, and other balance mechanisms can continue to perform at increased levels despite advancing age. We recently treated a 67-year-old woman whose balance problems led her to visit many different healthcare professionals for help; eventually she gave up and resigned herself to inactivity. Today after intense balance training, in a truly remarkable turnaround, she ice-skates semiprofessionally—an activity she had enjoyed with her husband when they were much younger.

ANATOMICAL AND HEALTH INFORMATION

The central nervous, vestibular, proprioceptive, and muscular systems play important roles in balance. Each provides your brain with a piece of information about the location of your body in space, which allows it to react when balance is altered.

Central Nervous System

The central nervous system, or brain and spinal cord, (see Figure 4.1) is your body's central command post. It coordinates, oversees, and responds to input from the rest of your body and ensures

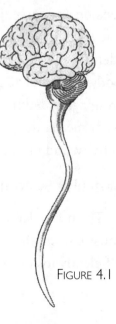

FIGURE 4.1

normal synchronized functioning of all systems. Each brain component plays a role in balance, but the cerebellum is most important. It coordinates the muscle activity over which you have voluntary control. The cerebellum receives and interprets motor and sensory information from the cerebrum, the vestibular system, and special receptors located in the muscles, tendons, joints, and skin.

Vestibular System

The vestibular system is located in the oval cavity of a bony structure called the labyrinth, which is part of your inner ear. It maintains stability during head or eye movement and provides your brain with information about your head position, so that your body can react accordingly.

Proprioceptors

Proprioceptors are nerve endings found in muscles, tendons, joints, and skin. Like the vestibular system, they communicate information about your body's movement and position. Muscle proprioceptors detect length changes within your muscles. Tendon proprioceptors communicate tension and force. Joint proprioceptors detect movement, joint position, and specific ranges of motion within the joint. Skin proprioceptors identify environmental changes and provide information about your body's postural alignment. Problems with proprioception may result from aging, failure to stretch regularly, habitually poor posture, faulty body mechanics, a lack of muscle use, a general decrease in physical activity, and increased stress and anxiety.

Muscular System

The muscular system also helps maintain balance. Without adequate muscle strength, your body will not be able to respond quickly and efficiently to correct its position when you lose your balance.

Connective Tissue Tightening

Your muscles, ligaments, or joints are all composed of connective tissue. They are prone to shortening or tightening as a result of several factors, including aging, failure to stretch regularly, habitually poor posture, and faulty body mechanics. Decreased flexibility of these structures can lead to balance problems.

Health-related Conditions

Many balance problems are the result of aging, but other conditions can also cause them. As you age, your neck discs may become thinner and prone to degenerative arthritic changes. As a result, you may hold your head in a position that compresses nearby blood vessels. Certain movements, such as turning to look over your shoulder, tilting your ear toward your shoulder, or moving your head back (like when you get your hair washed), or a combinations of these movements, may decrease blood flow in the vertebral arteries, possibly leading to dizziness or fainting. Blood flow to your head may also be impeded if the blood vessels in your neck that lead to your brain narrow as a result of arterial hardening (atherosclerotic disease). If you experience persistent dizziness, please consult your physician immediately.

Orthostatic or postural hypotension is abnormally low blood pressure that occurs when you move from lying to sitting or from sitting to standing. A quick change in position can lead to dizziness or light-headedness. This problem may be worse after you exercise or eat a large meal because more blood is shunted from your brain to other body parts. If the problem seems severe, consult your physician. If it is mild, the following guidance may help: Each time you move from lying down to sitting or from sitting to standing, stay still in the new position and breathe deeply for 30 seconds before you move any further. This will allow your blood pressure to reach its normal limits and should preclude any further light-headedness or dizziness.

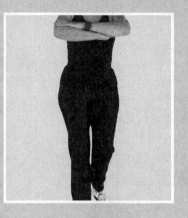 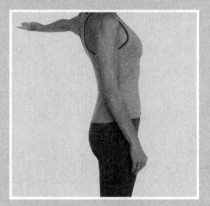 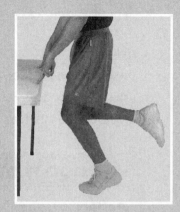

BALANCE ASSESSMENT

The following assessment will help you judge your balance. Take each test as described and record your results. After completing the tests, use the checklist to create your own balance profile and develop your most effective exercise program.

When you assess your balance, you will need to have someone assist you with some of the measurements. You should also have a friend or family member stand by, or stay near a stable surface or piece of furniture (a wall, counter, sturdy chair, or a dresser) in case you need support. As your balance improves, you can lessen your reliance on the support. Wear sneakers or other supportive, flat shoes.

To perform these tests, you'll need a 12-inch ruler, a yardstick, painter's tape, and a stopwatch or a clock with a second hand.

Caution: Consult your physician or physical therapist before you begin this program if you have any existing medical problems, if you currently experience any dizziness or major balance problems, or if you have recently fallen.

Note: Although the first 8 assessments in this section do not directly test your balance, they do assess factors that can significantly influence your equilibrium—blood flow to the head, blood pressure, flexibility, and muscle strength. The remaining 9 assessments focus on your ability to maintain your balance while you are static (still) or in motion.

BLOOD FLOW TO THE HEAD—A

Action: To test the flow of blood to your head, sit up straight in a chair. Turn your head to the right as far as you comfortably can (photo 1). Stay in this position for 30 seconds. Return to the starting position. Turn your head to the left as far as you comfortably can. Stay in this position for 30 seconds. Return to the starting position.

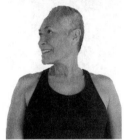

PHOTO 1

Score: Note whether or not you felt dizzy or light-headed.

Score:	Score:	Score:
Date:	Date:	Date:

Assessment: You should not experience any dizziness. If you did, check with your physician before proceeding with any exercise. With your doctor's approval, do exercise 1.

BLOOD FLOW TO THE HEAD—B

Action: To test the flow of blood to your head, sit up straight in a chair. Tilt your head back as far as possible (photo 1). Stay in this position for 30 seconds. Return to the starting position.

Score: Note whether or not you felt dizzy or light-headed.

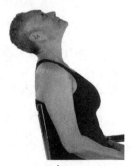

PHOTO 1

Score: Score: Score:

Date: Date: Date:

Assessment: You should not experience any dizziness. If you did, check with your physician before proceeding with any exercise. With your doctor's approval, do exercise 1.

BLOOD PRESSURE ADJUSTMENT—A

Action: To test your blood pressure adjustment, lie on a bed or other flat surface for 2 minutes (photo 1). Slowly sit up (photos 2 and 3). Lie down again for another 2 minutes. Now sit up quickly.

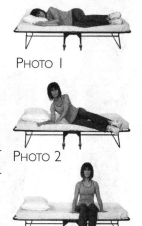

PHOTO 1

PHOTO 2

Score: Note whether or not you felt dizzy or light-headed.

Score: Score: Score:

Date: Date: Date:

Assessment: You should not experience any dizziness. If you did, check with your physician before proceeding with any exercise. With your doctor's approval, do exercise 2.

PHOTO 3

BLOOD PRESSURE ADJUSTMENT—B

Action: To test your blood pressure adjustment, sit up straight in a chair for 2 minutes. Slowly rise to a standing position. Sit down again for 2 minutes. Now stand up quickly.

Score: Note whether or not you felt dizzy or light-headed.

Score: Score: Score:

Date: Date: Date:

Assessment: You should not experience any dizziness. If you did, check with your physician before proceeding with any exercise. With your doctor's approval, do exercise 2.

FLEXIBILITY

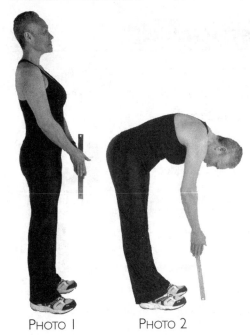

PHOTO 1   PHOTO 2

Action: To test your flexibility, warm up by walking for a few minutes. Stand up straight while holding a 12-inch ruler (photo 1). Slowly bend forward from the waist. Use the ruler to determine the distance between the tips of your middle fingers and the floor (photo 2).

Score: Record the distance between the tips of your middle fingers and the floor.

Score:	Score:	Score:
Date:	Date:	Date:

Assessment: If your fingertips were more than 2 inches from the floor, do the exercises in chapter 5.

MUSCLE STRENGTH—A

Action: To test your muscle strength, sit up straight in a chair. Do not lean back. Place your arms across your chest (photo 1). Time yourself as you rise to a complete stand (photo 2) and return to a seated position 10 times in a row.

Score: Record the time it took you to stand and sit 10 times.

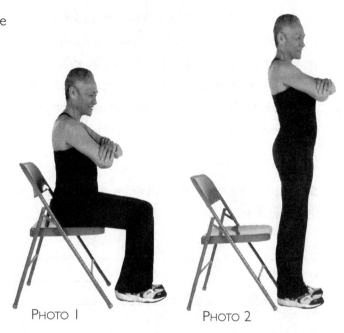

PHOTO 1   PHOTO 2

Score:	Score:	Score:
Date:	Date:	Date:

Assessment: Refer to Chart 1 in chapter 1 (page 11). If your time was slower than the norm for your age and gender, do exercise 2 in this chapter or Leg exercise 7 in chapter 3.

MUSCLE STRENGTH—B

Action: To test your muscle strength, stand on your right leg and lift your left leg off the floor; bend your left knee 90 degrees. If you have difficulty balancing, lightly place 1 or 2 fingers on a table, counter, or wall. Slowly and smoothly, rise up on the toes of your right foot (photo 1) and return to the starting position. Repeat 10 times or as many times as you can without discomfort.

Repeat the test, lifting your right leg.

Score: Record the number of times you were able to rise to your toes.

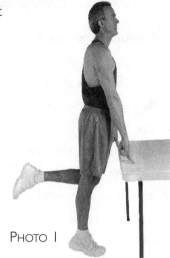

PHOTO 1

Right:	Right:	Right:
Left:	Left:	Left:
Date:	Date:	Date:

Assessment: If you were unable to complete 10 repetitions, do exercise 4.

MUSCLE STRENGTH—C

Action: To test your muscle strength, stand on your right leg and lift your left leg off the floor; bend your left knee 90 degrees. If you have difficulty balancing, lightly place 1 or 2 fingers on a table, counter, or wall. Slowly and smoothly, raise the toes of your right foot (photo 1). Repeat 5 times or as many times as you can without discomfort.

Repeat the test, lifting your right leg.

Score: Record the number of times you were able to perform the movement on each leg.

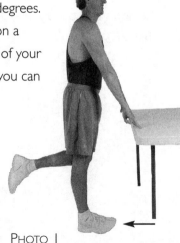

PHOTO 1

Right:	Right:	Right:
Left:	Left:	Left:
Date:	Date:	Date:

Assessment: If you were unable to complete this movement 5 times on each side, do Leg exercises 4 and 8 in chapter 3.

POSITION SENSE

Action: To test your position sense, stand up straight with your arms out to the side at shoulder height (photo 1). Slowly and smoothly, touch your right index fingertip to the end of your nose (photo 2). Return to the starting position. Touch your left index fingertip to the end of your nose, and then return to the starting position.

Score: Record whether or not you were able to complete the movement smoothly and accurately.

Score:	Score:	Score:
Date:	Date:	Date:

Assessment: If you were unable to complete the movement smoothly and accurately, do exercise 5.

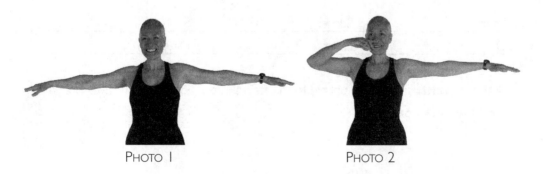

PHOTO 1   PHOTO 2

STATIC BALANCE—A

Action: To test your static balance, stand up straight with your feet together. Place your arms across your chest. Have someone time you as you maintain this position for up to 30 seconds or as long as is comfortable (photo 1).

Score: Record the time you were able to maintain this position.

Score: _____   Score: _____   Score: _____

Date: _____   Date: _____   Date: _____

Assessment: If you were unable to hold this position for 30 seconds, do exercise 6.

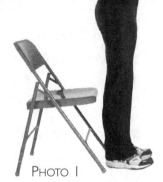

PHOTO 1

STATIC BALANCE—B

Action: To test your static balance, stand up straight with your feet together. Stay near a sturdy chair or counter in case you lose your balance. Place your arms across your chest. **Close your eyes.** Have someone time you as you maintain this position for up to 30 seconds or as long as is comfortable. Return to the starting position.

Score: Record the time you were able to maintain this position.

Score: _____   Score: _____   Score: _____

Date: _____   Date: _____   Date: _____

Assessment: If you were unable to maintain this position with your eyes closed for 30 seconds, do exercise 6.

STATIC BALANCE—C

Action: To test your static balance, stand up straight with your feet together. Stay near a sturdy chair or counter in case you lose your balance. Place your arms across your chest. Lift your left foot off the floor (photo 1). Have someone time you as you maintain this position for up to 30 seconds or as long as is comfortable. Return to the starting position.

Repeat the test, lifting your right leg.

Score: Record the time you were able to maintain the position on each leg.

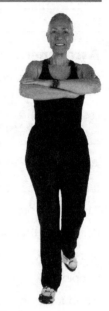

Right:	Right:	Right:
Left:	Left:	Left:
Date:	Date:	Date:

PHOTO 1

Assessment: If you were unable to hold the position on each side for 30 seconds, do exercise 6.

STATIC BALANCE—D

Action: To test your static balance, stand up straight with your feet together. Stay near a sturdy chair or counter in case you lose your balance. Place your arms across your chest. Lift your left foot off the floor. **Close your eyes.** Have someone time you as you maintain this position for up to 15 seconds or as long as is comfortable. Return to the starting position.

Repeat the test, lifting your right leg.

Score: Record the time you were able to maintain the position on each leg.

Right:	Right:	Right:
Left:	Left:	Left:
Date:	Date:	Date:

Assessment: : If you could not hold the position with your eyes closed on each side for 15 seconds, do exercise 6.

MOVING BALANCE—A

Action: To test your balance while moving forward, tape a yardstick horizontally on the wall at the height of your shoulders. (Use painter's tape, available at your local hardware store, to avoid damaging your wall.) Stand up straight with your right shoulder almost touching the wall. Raise your right arm to shoulder height so your fingertips are next to but not touching the end of the yardstick closest to you (photo 1). Keeping your shoulders parallel, bend at the waist and reach as far forward as possible without moving your feet (photo 2). Note the farthest point on the yardstick you were able to reach. Return to the starting position.

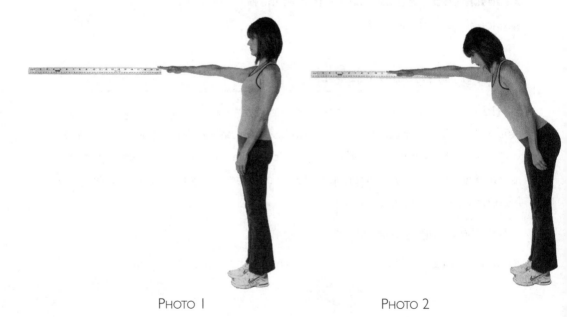

PHOTO 1   PHOTO 2

Score: Record the distance you were able to reach.

Score:	Score:	Score:
Date:	Date:	Date:

Assessment: If you were able to reach fewer than 6 inches, do exercises 3 and 7.

MOVING BALANCE—B

Action: To test your balance while moving backward, tape a yardstick horizontally on the wall at the height of your shoulders. Stand up straight with your right shoulder almost touching the wall. Raise your right arm to shoulder height so that your fingertips are next to but not touching the edge of the yardstick that is farthest away from you. Keeping

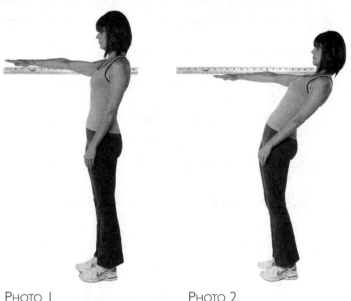

PHOTO 1   PHOTO 2

your shoulders parallel, and your arm as straight as possible, bend backward at the waist. Note the farthest point on the yardstick next to your fingertips. Return to the starting position.

Score: Record the distance you were able to reach.

Score:	Score:	Score:
Date:	Date:	Date:

Assessment: If you were able to reach fewer than 4-1/2 inches, do exercise 7.

MOVING BALANCE—C

Action: To test your balance while moving to the side, tape a yardstick horizontally on the wall at the height of your shoulders. Stand up straight with your back almost touching the wall. Raise your right arm to shoulder height and position yourself so that your right fingertips are touching the edge of the yardstick that is closest to you (photo 1). Keeping your shoulders parallel and your arms as straight as possible, bend at the waist and reach to the right as far as possible without moving your feet. Note the farthest point on the yardstick you were able to reach. Return to the starting position.

Repeat the test, using your left arm.

Score: Record the distances you were able to reach on each side.

Right:	Right:	Right:
Left:	Left:	Left:
Date:	Date:	Date:

Assessment: If you were unable to reach at least 6 inches, do exercises 3 and 7.

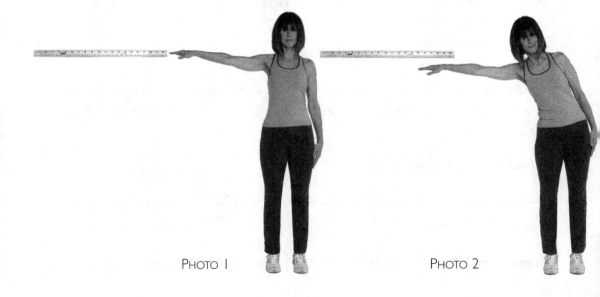

PHOTO 1   PHOTO 2

MOVING BALANCE (TANDEM WALKING)—D

Action: To test your balance while moving, stand at the end of an uncarpeted hallway that is at least 10 feet long. (If you must use a carpeted hallway, be sure the carpeting is a tight weave.) Placing 1 foot directly in front of the other, walk forward as if you are on a tightrope or balance beam for at least 10 feet, or as far as you can in this manner.

Score: : Record the distance you were able to walk.

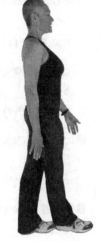

Score:	Score:	Score:
Date:	Date:	Date:

Assessment: If you were unable to walk 10 feet without stopping or stepping to the side, do exercise 8.

PHOTO 1

Wendy's Prescription for Balance

Wendy passed all the tests and decided not to set aside a special time to do any balance exercises, but she read the section on daily tips at the end of the chapter. She tries to stand on 1 leg while she brushes her teeth and walks on her heels and toes at least once a day.

James's Prescription for Balance

James took all the tests and performed poorly in static and moving balance. He could not stand on either leg with his eyes open for 30 seconds. He was only able to reach 4 inches with both hands on Moving Balance–A. James decided to perform 3 exercises: Forward Reaching (#3), One-Legged Stands (#6), and Dot Reaches (#7). He decided to do 3 repetitions of each exercise.

PRESCRIPTION FOR BALANCE

Date:_____

Blood Flow to the Head—A
  Score: _____
  Exercise(s) Needed: _____

Blood Flow to the Head—B
  Score: _____
  Exercise(s) Needed: _____

Blood Pressure Adjustment—A
  Score: _____
  Exercise(s) Needed: _____

Blood Pressure Adjustment—B
  Score: _____
  Exercise(s) Needed: _____

Flexibility
  Distance: _____
  Exercise(s) Needed: _____

Muscle Strength—A
  Time: _____
  Exercise(s) Needed: _____

Muscle Strength—B
  Number on right: _____
  Number on left: _____
  Exercise(s) Needed: _____

Muscle Strength—C
  Number on right: _____
  Number on left: _____
  Exercise(s) Needed: _____

Position Sense
  Score: _____
  Exercise(s) Needed: _____

Static Balance—A
  Time: _____
  Exercise(s) Needed: _____

Static Balance—B
  Time: _____
  Exercise(s) Needed: _____

Static Balance—C
  Time on right: _____
  Time on left: _____
  Exercise(s) Needed: _____

Static Balance—D
  Time on right: _____
  Time on left: _____
  Exercise(s) Needed: _____

Moving Balance—A
  Distance: _____
  Exercise(s) Needed: _____

Moving Balance—B
  Distance: _____
  Exercise(s) Needed: _____

Moving Balance—C
  Distance on right: _____
  Distance on left: _____
  Exercise(s) Needed: _____

Moving Balance (Tandem Walking)—D
  Distance: _____
  Exercise(s) Needed: _____

(Make a copy for your personal use)

8 GREAT EXERCISES FOR BALANCE

#1 Head Turns

#2 Sit-to-Stands

#3 Forward Reaching

#4 Heel-Toe Walking

#5 Finger-to-Nose

#6 One-Legged Stands

#7 Dot Reaches

#8 Tandem Walking

Note: Exercises #2, #5, and #8 appear in this book both as assessments and as exercises. Perfecting the skills used to perform these actions is especially important to your physical fitness. If you are assigned the same exercise more than once, you only need to do the repetitions from 1 chapter, not both.

#1 ■ Head Turns

Why this exercise? This exercise will communicate information to your brain about your body's position in space and improve the movement of your head. It is particularly important if you tend to keep your head in 1 position for long periods of time, failing to move it through the full range of motion.

1. Sit up straight in a supportive chair. Tuck in your chin (photo 1).

2. Turn your head to the right and then to the left 5 times, gradually increasing your speed (photo 2).

3. Repeat this movement 3 times.

4. Lower your chin to your chest and then raise it toward the ceiling, gradually increasing your speed (photo 3).

5. Repeat this movement 3 times.

6. Perform this exercise once or twice a day.

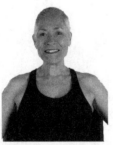
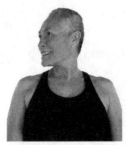
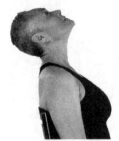

Photo 1   Photo 2   Photo 3

#2 ■ Sit-to-Stands

Why this exercise? This exercise will help your body adjust when you change position. If you are sedentary, spending hours in the same position, your sense of balance will be affected. This exercise will help you avoid feeling dizzy when you stand up suddenly. It will also strengthen the muscles in your buttocks and lower legs.

1. Sit up straight in a supportive chair. Do not lean back. Place your arms across your chest (photo 1).

2. Rise to a complete stand (photo 2) and return to a seated position as quickly as possible. Do not use your arms.

3. Repeat this movement 3 times in a row initially, and build to 10 times as you get stronger.

4. Perform this exercise once or twice a day.

Note: If you do not have the strength to perform this exercise without using your arms, you may use them initially. As you get stronger, gradually lessen the use of your arms.

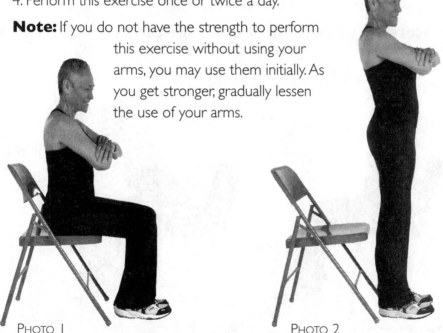

PHOTO 1   PHOTO 2

#3 ■ Forward Reaching

Why this exercise? This exercise will improve your stability. By stressing its limits, you can learn to move more comfortably in all directions without fear of losing your balance. If you tend to hold your trunk in 1 position for long periods, this exercise will improve your range of motion.

1. Sit in a supportive chair. Keeping your arms straight, raise them in front of you to shoulder height (photo 1).

2. Keeping your back and arms as straight as possible and your shoulders parallel, reach forward as far as you can (photo 2). Breathe deeply and hold this position for 10 seconds.

3. Return to the starting position.

4. Repeat this movement 1 to 3 times.

5. Perform this exercise once or twice a day.

Note: If you have medium to severe osteoporosis, do not do this exercise.

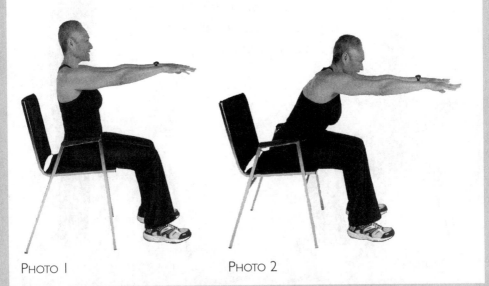

PHOTO 1   PHOTO 2

#4 ■ Heel-Toe Walking

Why this exercise? This exercise will improve your coordination and strengthen your leg and trunk muscles. Perform this exercise in a hallway or other area where you can walk at least 10 feet without encountering any obstructions. The area should be uncarpeted or have firm flooring, such as wood, vinyl or ceramic tile, laminate, linoleum, or low-pile or flat-weave carpet.

1. Stand up straight. Lift your toes and the balls of your feet off the floor, so that you are balanced on your heels.

2. Walk 10 steps on your heels while keeping your body as straight as possible (photo 1).

3. Return to the starting position. Rise onto your toes. Walk 10 steps on your toes, keeping your body as straight as possible (photo 2).

4. Repeat these movements 1 to 3 times.

5. Perform this exercise once or twice a day.

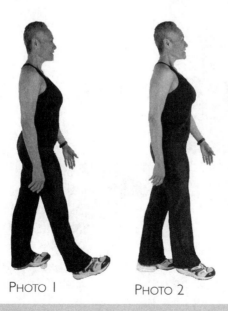

PHOTO 1   PHOTO 2

#5 ■ Finger-to-Nose

Why this exercise? This exercise will improve your hand and arm coordination and help you move more precisely.

1. Stand up straight or sit in a supportive chair. Raise your arms out to the side at shoulder height (photo 1).

2. Slowly and smoothly touch your right index fingertip to the end of your nose (photo 2).

3. Return to the starting position.

4. Repeat this movement 3 times.

5. Return to the starting position. Touch your left index fingertip to your nose.

6. Repeat this movement 3 times.

7. Perform this exercise once or twice a day.

8. To increase the difficulty, close your eyes.

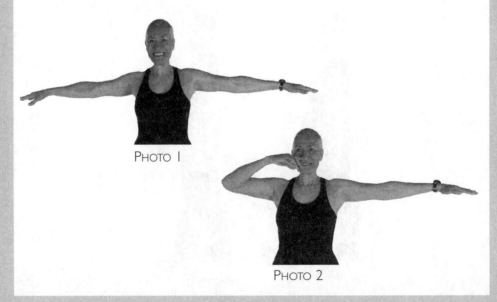

PHOTO 1

PHOTO 2

#6 ■ One-Legged Stands

Why this exercise? This exercise will increase the limits of your stability, which will lessen your risk of losing your balance. It will also strengthen your legs.

1. Stand up straight behind a sturdy chair or by a counter in case you lose your balance. Keeping your arms straight, raise them in front of you to shoulder height (photo 1).

2. Bend your left knee and lift your left foot off the floor (photo 2). Maintain this position for 30 seconds. Lower your left foot to the floor.

3. Bend your right knee and lift your right foot off the floor. Maintain this position for 30 seconds.

4. Repeat this movement 3 times on each side.

5. Perform this exercise once or twice a day.

6. To increase the difficulty, close your eyes.

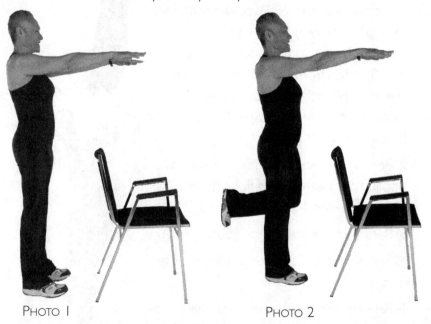

PHOTO 1   PHOTO 2

#7 ■ Dot Reaches

Why this exercise? This exercise will help you control your balance when you reach. Keep your feet close together to make it more challenging. Place 2 dots on the wall: 1 at the height of your shoulder and another at the height of the top of your head. Now place 2 additional dots at the same height on either side of the original 2, spacing them 5 inches apart. When you are done, you should have 6 dots, in 2 rows of 3, spaced 5 inches apart. (You can use the small circular stickers available in office supply stores, bits of painter's tape, or pencil marks.)

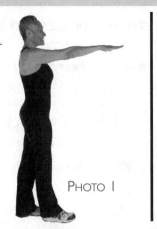

PHOTO 1

1. Stand up straight 3 feet away from the wall on which you've placed the dots. Face the wall and extend your right arm at shoulder height so that your fingertips are 4 to 8 inches from the dots. Keep your arm straight and your feet parallel and hip-width apart; move your right foot slightly in front of your left (photo 1).

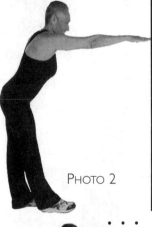

PHOTO 2

2. Bend at the waist and lean forward. Do not lift your heels off the floor (photo 2). Touch each dot 10 times (photo 3).

3. Return to the starting position.

4. Repeat these movements using your left arm.

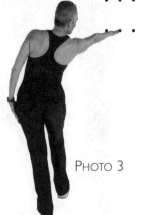

PHOTO 3

5. Perform this exercise once or twice a day.

#8 ■ Tandem Walking

Why this exercise? This exercise will improve your coordination. It will also strengthen your leg and trunk muscles. Perform this exercise in a hallway or other area where you can walk at least 10 feet without encountering any obstructions. The area should be uncarpeted or have firm flooring, such as wood, vinyl or ceramic tile, laminate, linoleum, or low-pile or flat-weave carpet.

1. Stand up straight at the end of the hallway. Keep your stomach muscles tight and your chin tucked in.

2. Placing 1 foot directly in front of the other, walk forward as if you were on a tightrope or balance beam for about 10 feet (photo 1).

3. Repeat this activity 1 to 3 times.

4. Perform this exercise once or twice a day, or whenever you walk down a long hallway.

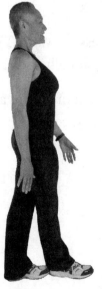

PHOTO 1

DAILY TIPS AND ENERGIZING IDEAS

This section includes easy-to-do tasks, modifications to daily activities, and hints to enhance and reinforce the exercises in your balance program. Place little notes to yourself everywhere you tend to look during the day as reminders to do them from time to time.

AT HOME AND WORK

■ When you walk down a hallway, swing your arms or turn your head left and right to challenge your balance.

■ Stand on 1 leg while you are on the phone or watching TV. For an additional challenge, close your eyes.

■ While you dust, slowly move from 1 piece of furniture to the next without taking a break.

■ While you sit at your desk or watch TV, periodically turn your head from side-to-side, gradually increasing your range of motion.

■ When you wait near a wall or ride in an elevator, practice dot reaches (without the dots, of course).

GROOMING AND PREPARING MEALS

■ While you brush your teeth or wash dishes, balance on your toes. Lower your heels. Then balance on your heels. Do these movements while you stand on 1 leg.

■ When you stand at the stove, raise and lower your heels as quickly as possible.

■ While you dress, turn your head from side-to-side after you put on each piece of clothing.

IN THE GYM

■ As you move from 1 piece of equipment to another, walk on your toes or on your heels, or tandem walk.

■ When you use a treadmill, elliptical machine, or stepper, try to avoid using the handrails. You will get a better workout and improve your balance.

■ When you use equipment, stand or sit straight, tuck in your chin, bring your shoulders back and slightly down, and tighten your abdominals.

■ Take Tai Chi classes.

■ Challenge your balance frequently. Balance on 1 leg as you lift weights with your arms. Stand or balance on all fours on a BOSU (Both Sides Up Balance Trainer) or on foam pads. The more your balance is challenged, the more it will improve.

Tai Chi and Balance?

Tai Chi (sometimes spelled t'ai chi, tai ji, or tai qi) is one of the Chinese martial arts. Its name, loosely translated, means "great internal energy," and the practice has always been associated with balance, relaxation, and healing. Numerous studies have shown the benefits of practicing Tai Chi as part of a balance program. Continued practice of its movement sequences can improve ease and grace of movement and balance. The balance components of Tai Chi include:

- Performing continuous movements slowly.
- Keeping your knees slightly bent and your weight moving from 1 leg to the other.
- Maintaining well aligned posture while moving slowly.
- Combining rotational movements of the arms, legs, and trunk.

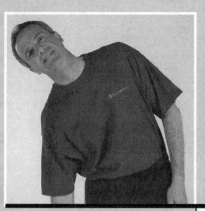

Chapter 5

Flexibility

Can a Coke Bottle Make You More Flexible?

Here's a good way to keep your legs and feet flexible while sitting for a long time. Get an old-fashioned 8-ounce glass Coca-Cola bottle, place it under your foot, and roll it back and forth. Believe it or not, this will keep your legs and feet from getting stiff.

Many years ago a patient told one of us about this technique. At the time, this style of bottle was no longer produced, but the patient insisted this was what had to be used because of its shape; the curve of the bottle fits a foot perfectly and prevents it from slipping.

But where to get this exact bottle? The author placed a call to Coca-Cola's headquarters in Atlanta and was surprised and delighted to be put through to a vice-president. He listened intently and then said that as the result of an old football injury, his knee would stiffen whenever he sat at his desk for long periods of time. The executive requested information about the exercise and said he would try it. "If it relieves the stiffness in my knee," he promised, "I'll send you a case of bottles."

Several months later a deliveryman arrived at the clinic with 6 cases of Coca-Cola in the 8-ounce bottles and a thank-you note.

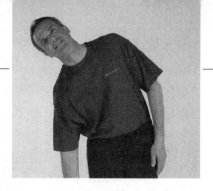

*You are aging when your actions
creak louder than your words.*

—MILTON BERLE

Flexibility is an often-neglected part of physical fitness. Being limber gives you the freedom to move, whether it's bending over to tie your shoes, reaching up to retrieve something from a high shelf, or picking up items more easily. Flexibility is associated with your joints and connective tissue as well as your muscles. You should approach flexibility training exercises in the same way you approach aerobic conditioning or strength training—you must do them regularly since they are an important part of total fitness, particularly as you age.

Susan, 59, could swear that the mailbox had moved. For 20 years she had been looking over her shoulder as she backed down the driveway, using that mailbox to line up her car. Lately she couldn't quite swivel her head around far enough to find her landmark. Of course, she knew her mailbox hadn't migrated—not even an inch. Her ability to turn her head had changed.

PROPER FLEXIBILITY

Flexibility is simply the ability of body parts to bend without breaking, or in other words, the pliability of the body. Flexibility allows your joints to bend repeatedly without any damage or injury.

The connections between your bones are called joints (Figure 5.1); every joint has a specific range of motion. For example, you should be able to raise your arms overhead 180 degrees, bend your elbow 145 degrees, tilt your neck 45 degrees to the side, arch your back 30 degrees, rotate your hip 45 degrees, and extend your knee 0 degrees (in a straight line). Staying limber helps you balance and perform daily activities more comfortably. Flexibility helps reduce muscle tension, improve

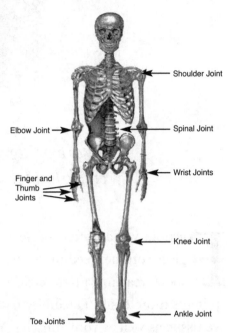

FIGURE 5.1

coordination, prevent injuries, develop body awareness, and even promote good circulation.

FLEXIBILITY CHANGES

Flexibility decreases as a result of inactivity and changes in the collagen structures of the body. Collagen is a protein found in connective tissue—tendons, ligaments, joint capsules, coverings around the muscles, and skin. As you age, collagen tends to stick together, the linings of your joints thicken, and the fibrous tissue surrounding your joints increases. You may also experience degeneration of the ligaments surrounding your joints.

As a result, you may have a noticeable loss of elasticity and flexibility—a decline in your ability to move fluidly and precisely, a decrease in your range of motion, and possibly even conditions such as contractures (permanent shortening of muscles or tendons) or ankylosis (bone fusing in your joints). If you regularly stretch your muscles, ligaments, and joint capsules, you may avoid some of these problems and stay flexible.

ANATOMICAL AND HEALTH INFORMATION

Joints

There are many different types of joints, including hinged (finger and elbow), modified hinge (knee), ball and socket (hip, shoulder), and gliding (spine). Almost all joints consist of a cartilage lining, a capsule, ligaments, and a membrane.

The cartilage lining allows the joint to move smoothly and absorbs some of the shock transmitted during movement. The capsule, which consists of connective tissue, helps stabilize the joint. Ligaments, which are also made of connective tissue, provide support for the joint. Many joints also have a membrane that secretes fluid to facilitate movement.

Connective Tissue

Connective tissue plays an enormous role in how loose or tight your body is. It stretches in 2 ways: elastic and plastic.

Elastic stretch occurs when a structure is elongated by an external force; when the force is released the structure returns to its original position. An easy example is a new rubber band: stretch it as far as you can before it breaks and then release it. It will snap back to its original position.

Plastic stretch occurs when a structure is stretched or elongated by an external force over a prolonged period of time; when the force is released, the structure remains stretched. For example, if you wrap a rubber band around a box and leave the box in a closet for a long time, the rubber band will remain permanently stretched once it has been removed from the box.

You can experience either of these when you stretch your hamstring muscles. Sit with your leg extended in front of you. If you try to reach for your toes by bouncing, you will be performing an elastic stretch. If you reach for your toes in a slow, gentle fashion and hold the position for 30 to 60 seconds, you will get a good plastic stretch.

Collagen tissue is a thick but flexible material and will respond to elastic or plastic stretch. To increase your flexibility and avoid injury, you need to hold your stretches for longer periods of time. Warming up first will also improve the quality of your stretching and lower your chance of injury. Bouncing while stretching is usually not recommended.

Health-related Conditions

Osteoarthritis, rheumatoid arthritis, and polymyalgia rheumatica are diseases that affect the joints and their surrounding muscles, making it painful to move and often leading to a cycle of decreased motion and increased stiffness. After appropriate treatment, a patient should return to a program of increasing physical activity to enhance fitness and functional ability.

Osteoarthritis

Osteoarthritis (OA) is a degeneration of the joints characterized by the wearing away of the cartilage that covers the ends of bones. OA is divided into 2 types: primary and secondary. Primary osteoarthritis is the result of wear and tear on your joints as you age. There are many potential causes or risk factors associated with the development of secondary osteoarthritis, including genetic defects, trauma to or overuse of a joint, and diseases such as diabetes, obesity, inflammatory joint diseases, sickle cell disease, and Paget disease (a destructive bone disease).

Osteoarthritis is the most common joint disease. X-rays reveal evidence of OA in one-third of people over 35; this number increases to more than 80 percent in people over age 70. It is the leading cause of disability in people over 65.

OA increases bone formation at the edges of the joint and causes degenerative changes in the membrane surrounding the joint. It usually begins with a slow increase in pain, particularly in joints that have been subjected to large amounts of stress over the years, such as the hips, knees, lower spine, neck, toes, and fingers. Initially, the pain is often intermittent, but it may become constant. Eventually a person afflicted with OA may develop swollen joints and experience limited mobility. To diagnose OA, a doctor takes a history and obtains x-rays of the joint(s) involved; he may also take fluid out of the joint for analysis.

Treatment of osteoarthritis can include rest, medication, exercise, and surgery. If your OA is moderate to severe, please see a physical therapist before beginning any exercise program. Physical therapists may use exercises, manual techniques (such as range of motion exercises and soft tissue massage) and modalities (such as heat, ice, electricity, and sound) to help you get started. It is not true that you must learn to live with OA. There are always new methods and treatments. Seek an appropriate healthcare provider who offers a wide range of interventions for joint changes associated with osteoarthritis.

Osteoarthritis can also be treated by joint replacement surgery, particularly if the problem is located in the hip or knee joints. Shoulder, elbow, wrist, finger, and ankle joint replacements are also done, but are not as common.

No matter what the treatment, exercise is always beneficial. Physical therapy is one of the best and safest treatments for OA. If your condition is mild—or if your physical therapist has approved it—the exercises in this chapter, as well as those in chapters 2 and 3, will be helpful.

Rheumatoid Arthritis

Rheumatoid arthritis (RA) is a systemic disease resulting in an inflammation of connective tissues throughout the body. The exact cause is unknown, but the immune system seems to play an important role. Researchers have also indicated that there may be a genetic link and infection may be a triggering factor. RA also leads to inflammation of the membrane around the joint, destruction of the joint cartilage, capsule, and muscles, and eventually total immobility or fusion of the joint. RA usually begins earlier in life than osteoarthritis, often appearing in individuals between the ages of 20 and 40. It is initially characterized by minimal symptoms of joint pain and swelling and later by intense inflammation of the small joints of the hands, feet, and wrists. As the disease progresses, the elbows, shoulders, knees, and hips can become affected. Other effects include fatigue, depression, loss of appetite, and significant stiffness lasting longer than an hour after waking. To diagnose RA, a doctor often examines the patient's blood to check for high erythrosedimentation rate (ESR) and rheumatoid factor (RF).

Patients with RA may be treated with medication (ranging from aspirin or nonsteroidal anti-inflammatory drugs to antibiotics and antimetabolite agents), physical therapy, an individualized exercise program, an energy conservation program, and appropriate assistive devices. Exercises aimed at improving posture, strength, and balance (such as those in chapters 2, 3, and 4) can also be beneficial. Joint replacement surgery is another treatment option, particularly for the hip, knee, and shoulder joints. If you have RA, please see a physical therapist before beginning an exercise program.

Polymyalgia Rheumatica

Polymyalgia rheumatica (PMR) is an arthritic disease primarily found in people—mostly Caucasian women—50 years and older. The exact cause is unknown, but it is believed to be associated with an inflammation of the blood vessels. PMR is characterized by tender, swollen joints and painful, stiff muscles in the hips and shoulders. Though PMR usually gets better within 5 years of onset, it may become so severe that it leads to immobility and loss of function. Without treatment, a person with PMR may experience significant discomfort and may have complications that affect organs, including the kidneys and liver. This disease may even cause blindness. To diagnose PMR, a doctor will take a history, perform an examination, and order laboratory tests that may include measurement of the electric current in the muscles, muscle biopsy, and analysis of the erthrocyte sedimentation rate (ESR).

Treatment usually consists of a low dose of corticosteroids. Physical therapy can be helpful for decreasing pain, increasing motion of the joints affected, and regaining strength that may have been lost. Physical therapy may include strengthening and range of motion exercises, protection of body parts, instruction in how to perform activities of daily living, relaxation techniques, assistive devices, and modalities (e.g., heat, cold).

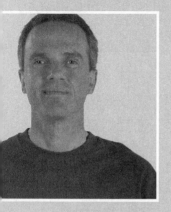
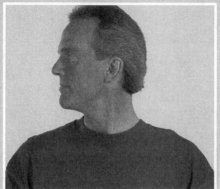
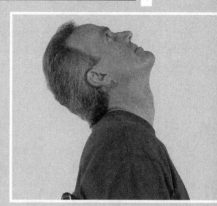

FLEXIBILITY ASSESSMENT

The following assessment will help you judge your flexibility. Take each test as described and record your results. After completing the tests, use the checklist to create your own flexibility profile and develop your most effective exercise program.

If you have particular concerns about your flexibility, see a physical therapist; he or she can devise a program that will be most effective for you.

To perform these tests, you'll need a 12-inch ruler and a yardstick. Wear sneakers or other flat shoes. You will need to have someone assist you with some of the measurements.

Caution: Consult your physician or physical therapist before you begin this program if you have any existing medical or back problems or have experienced joint pain for a period of time.

NECK FLEXION

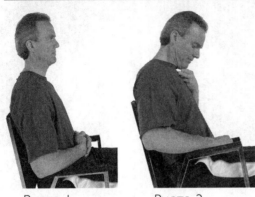

PHOTO 1   PHOTO 2

Action: To test your ability to bring your chin to your chest, sit up straight in an armchair. Tighten your stomach muscles and tuck in your chin. Place your arms on the armrests (photo 1). Bring your chin to your chest. Keep your mouth closed and do not move your upper body. Use your fingers to measure the distance between your chin and your chest (photo 2). Your chin should almost touch your chest and be no more than 2 fingers breadth away from your chest.

Score: Record the number of fingers between your chin and your chest.

Score: _____   Score: _____   Score: _____

Date: _____   Date: _____   Date: _____

Assessment: If you could fit more than 2 fingers between your chin and your chest, do exercise 2.

NECK EXTENSION

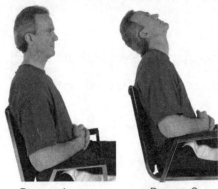

PHOTO 1   PHOTO 2

Action: To test your ability to tilt your head back, sit up straight in an armchair. Tighten your stomach muscles and tuck in your chin. Place your arms on the armrests (photo 1). Tilt your head back and look at the ceiling. Keep your mouth closed (photo 2). Have someone check your position; your head should be almost parallel to the floor. You should be able to look at the ceiling without moving your upper body.

Score: Record the position of your head.

Score:	Score:	Score:
Date:	Date:	Date:

Assessment: If you could not tilt your head all the way back, do exercise 7.

NECK ROTATION

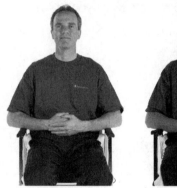

PHOTO 1

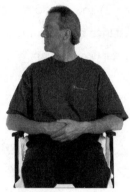

PHOTO 2

Action: To test your neck rotation, sit up straight in an armchair. Tighten your stomach muscles and tuck in your chin. Place your arms on the armrests (photo 1). Keep your shoulders and shoulder blades lowered and steady. Turn your head as far to the right as you comfortably can. Keep your mouth closed (photo 2). Your chin should be almost over your shoulder, and you should be able to see part of the wall behind you. Return to the starting position.

Repeat this test, turning to the left.

Score: Record the position of your chin in relation to your shoulder.

Right:	Right:	Right:
Left:	Left:	Left:
Date:	Date:	Date:

Assessment: If you were not able to move your chin almost over your shoulder, do exercise 6.

NECK LATERAL FLEXION

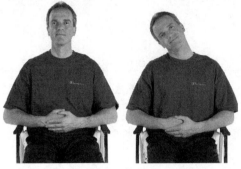

PHOTO 1   PHOTO 2

Action: To test your ability to tilt your head to the side, sit up straight in an armchair. Tighten your stomach muscles and tuck in your chin. Place your arms on the armrests (photo 1). Keep your shoulders and shoulder blades lowered and steady.

Tilt your head to the right, bringing your right earlobe toward your right shoulder. Look straight ahead and do not turn your head or move your left shoulder (photo 2). You should be able to tilt your head between one-third and one-half the distance between the starting position of your head and your shoulder. Return to the starting position.

Repeat this test on the left.

Score: Record the position of your head.

Right:	Right:	Right:
Left:	Left:	Left:
Date:	Date:	Date:

Assessment: If you were unable to tilt your head one-third of the distance between your shoulder and the starting position of your head, do exercise 1.

SHOULDER FLEXIBILITY

Action: To test the flexibility of your shoulders, sit up straight in a chair. Do not lean back against the backrest. Tighten your stomach muscles and tuck in your chin.

Move your right hand, palm facing down, up and over your right shoulder until it is touching your right shoulder blade.

Move your left hand, palm facing out, behind and up your back (photo 1).

Have someone measure the distance between the tips of your middle fingers (photo 2). It's normal for that distance to be between 1 and 2 inches; there should be no more than 2 inches between your middle fingers. Return to the starting position.

Repeat this test by reversing the positions of your arms.

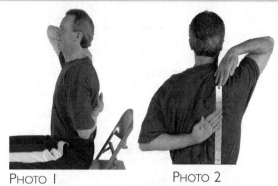

PHOTO 1   PHOTO 2

Score: Record the distance on each side.

Right:	Right:	Right:
Left:	Left:	Left:
Date:	Date:	Date:

Assessment: If the distance between your middle fingers was greater than 2 inches, do exercises 3 and 4.

HAND FLEXIBILITY

Action: To test the flexibility of your hands, stand up straight about 6 inches from a table or desk.

Place your palms flat down on the table, with your arms shoulder-width apart. Spread your fingers as far apart as possible (photo 1). Lock your elbows and lean forward, keeping your hands flat on the table (photo 2). Have someone measure how far your forearms moved forward. You should be able to move your forearms 2 to 4 inches forward without feeling a major pull in the muscles of your hands or forearms.

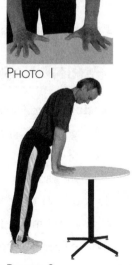

PHOTO 1

Score: Record the distance you were able to move your forearms.

PHOTO 2

Score:	Score:	Score:
Date:	Date:	Date:

Assessment: If you were unable to move your forearms 2 to 4 inches or felt a pulling sensation in your hand or forearms, do exercise 7.

SPINE FLEXION

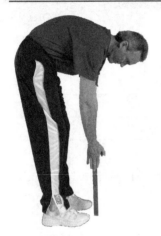

Action: To test your ability to bend over, stand up straight while holding a 12-inch ruler. Tighten your stomach muscles and tuck in your chin. Slowly bend forward from the waist and rest the end of the ruler on the floor. Slide your hands down the ruler as far as comfortably possible. Use the ruler to determine the distance between the tips of your middle fingers and the floor. Your fingertips should be no more than 2 inches from the floor.

Score: Record the distance between the tips of your middle fingers and the floor.

Score:	Score:	Score:
Date:	Date:	Date:

Assessment: If your fingertips were more than 2 inches from the floor, do exercise 8.

SPINE LATERAL FLEXION

Action: To test your ability to bend to the side, stand up straight, holding a yardstick in your right hand (photo 1). Tighten your stomach muscles and tuck in your chin. Keeping your knees straight and your body aligned, bend to the right and slide your right hand down the yardstick as far as comfortably possible. Think of your body as a pendulum; don't twist or move forward. Use the yardstick to measure the distance between the tip of your right middle finger and the floor (photo 2). The distance between your fingertip and the floor depends on your spinal flexibility and your height but it should be between

15 and 25 inches. Lower numbers are more appropriate for shorter people, higher for taller. You should be able to lean the same distance on each side. Return to the starting position.

Repeat this test on the left.

Score: Record the distance on each side.

Right:	Right:	Right:
Left:	Left:	Left:
Date:	Date:	Date:

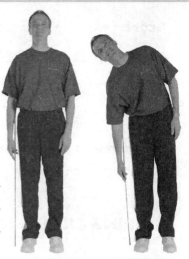

PHOTO 1   PHOTO 2

Assessment: If you were unable to lean between 15 and 25 inches from the floor or if you felt tighter on one side than the other, do exercise 1.

SPINE ROTATION

Action: To test your ability to twist your spine, lie on your back on the floor. Bend your knees, keeping your legs together and your feet close to your buttocks. Tighten your stomach muscles and tuck in your chin. Straighten your arms and stretch them out flat against the floor at shoulder height with your palms facing down (photo 1). Lower your legs to the right, keeping them together and your knees bent. Have someone measure the distance between the bottom of your right knee and the floor (photo 2). You should be able to almost touch the floor with your knee. Return to the starting position.

Repeat this test on the left.

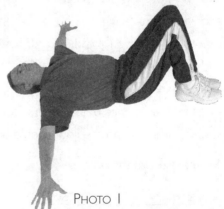

PHOTO 1

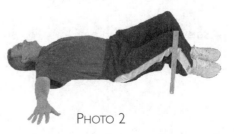

PHOTO 2

Score: Record the distances on each side.

Right:	Right:	Right:
Left:	Left:	Left:
Date:	Date:	Date:

Assessment: If you could not lower your legs close to the floor on both sides or if you felt tighter on one side than the other, do exercise 6.

SPINE EXTENSION

Action: Lie on your stomach on the floor. Tighten your stomach muscles and tuck in your chin. Keep your arms and hands flat on the floor with your fingers spread and your palms facing down (photo 1). Raise your head and upper body off the floor. Look down. Have someone

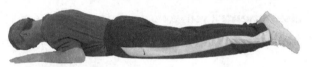

PHOTO 1

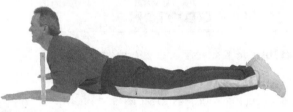

PHOTO 2

measure the distance between your collarbones and the floor. The distance between your collarbones and the floor should be 10 to 12 inches.

Score: Record the distance.

Score:	Score:	Score
Date:	Date:	Date:

Assessment: Both men and women should be able to lift at least 10 to 12 inches. If you could not, do exercise 7.

HIP FLEXION, ABDUCTION, AND ROTATION

Action: To test
the flexibility of your
hips, sit up straight
on the floor. Bend
your knees so that
the soles of your
feet touch. Tighten
your stomach mus-
cles and tuck in your
chin (photo 1). Using

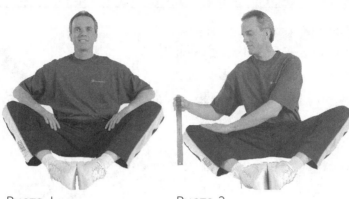

PHOTO 1   PHOTO 2

your left hand, gently press your right thigh down toward the floor. With a ruler in
your right hand, measure the distance between the floor and the bottom of your
right knee (photo 2). There should be no more than 6 inches between the bottom of
your knee and the floor. Return to the starting position.

Repeat this test on the left.

Score: Record the distance on each side.

Right:	Right:	Right:
Left:	Left:	Left:
Date:	Date:	Date:

Assessment: If the distance between the bottom of your knee and the floor was
greater than 6 inches or if 1 side was tighter than the other, do exercise 2.

HIP EXTENSION

Action: To test your ability to stretch your leg backward, lie on your back with your knees bent and your feet flat on the floor (photo 1). Wrap your hands under your right thigh and pull your right knee toward your chest. Straighten your left leg. Your left leg should be absolutely straight with the heel and the back of the calf flat on the floor; if it is not, have someone measure the distance between your left heel and the floor (photo 2). Return to the starting position.

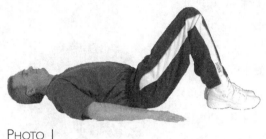

PHOTO 1

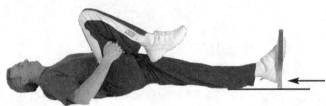

PHOTO 2

Repeat this test by reversing the positions of your legs.

Score: Record the distance on each side.

Right:	Right:	Right:
Left:	Left:	Left:
Date:	Date:	Date:

Assessment: If the calf and heel of your extended leg did not touch the floor and your knee was not straight, do exercise 5.

CALF FLEXIBILITY

Action: To test the flexibility of your calves, stand up straight facing a wall. Place your hands on the wall for support, the toes of your right foot at the edge of the wall, and your left foot back approximately 20 inches. Gently bend your right leg so that the knee is directly above the ankle (photo 1). The heel of

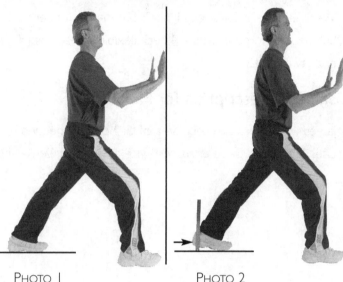

PHOTO 1   PHOTO 2

your left leg should stay flat on the floor as you bend your right knee. If your heel is not flat on the ground, have someone measure the distance between your left heel and the floor (photo 2). Return to the starting position.

Repeat this test by reversing the positions of your legs.

Score: Record the distance on each side.

Right:	Right:	Right:
Left:	Left:	Left:
Date:	Date:	Date:

Assessment: If the heel of your back leg does not stay on the floor as you bend your front knee, do exercise 8.

Wendy's Prescription for Flexibility

Wendy's neck flexibility was limited, but the rest of her body was extremely flexible. She decided to perform the 4 neck flexibility exercises (#1, #2, #6, and #7) 3 times each, twice a day.

James's Prescription for Flexibility

James was inflexible in each area of his body. He needed to do all 8 stretching exercises. He will do these exercises twice a day for 8 weeks and then retest himself.

PRESCRIPTION FOR FLEXIBILITY

Date:_____

Neck Flexion
Number of fingers: _____
Exercise(s) Needed: _____

Neck Extension
Position: _____
Exercise(s) Needed: _____

Neck Rotation
Position on right: _____
Position on left: _____
Exercise(s) Needed: _____

Neck Lateral Flexion
Position on right: _____
Position on left: _____
Exercise(s) Needed: _____

Shoulder Flexibility
Distance on right: _____
Distance on left: _____
Exercise(s) Needed: _____

Hand Flexibility
Distance: _____
Exercise(s) Needed: _____

Spine Flexion
Distance: _____
Exercise(s) Needed: _____

Spine Lateral Flexion

Distance on right: _____

Distance on left: _____

Exercise(s) Needed: _____

Spine Rotation

Distance on right: _____

Distance on left: _____

Exercise(s) Needed: _____

Spine Extension

Distance: _____

Exercise(s) Needed: _____

Hip Flexion, Abduction, and Rotation

Distance on right: _____

Distance on left: _____

Exercise(s) Needed: _____

Hip Extension

Distance on right: _____

Distance on left: _____

Exercise(s) Needed: _____

Calf Flexibility

Distance on right: _____

Distance on left: _____

Exercise(s) Needed: _____

(Make a copy for your personal use)

8 GREAT EXERCISES FOR FLEXIBILITY

#1 Neck Lateral Flexions

#2 Neck/Trunk Flexions and Hip Flexions/
Abductions/External Rotations

#3 "W" Wall Stretches

#4 Shoulder Combined Movements

#5 Spine Flexions/Hip Flexions and Extensions

#6 Spine and Neck Rotations

#7 Spine Extensions

#8 Leg Stretches

SAFE STRETCHING

- Always warm up before you stretch.
- It's normal to feel mild discomfort, mild tension, or a mild pulling sensation, but stretching should never cause pain.
- Relax as you hold a stretch; the feeling of tension should subside. When it does, stretch slightly further until you feel a mild tension. Hold this position for 30 to 60 seconds.
- Never bounce—a stretch should be slow and steady.
- Avoid locking your joints; they should remain soft.
- Breathe deeply, slowly, and rhythmically during the stretch.
- Focus on the body part you are stretching.
- Stretch regularly.

#1 ■ Neck Lateral Flexions

Why this exercise? This exercise will loosen the muscles in the sides of your neck and spine, which may be tight if you have a sedentary job. It will make it easier to tilt your head to the side, or turn your head as you lean to the side.

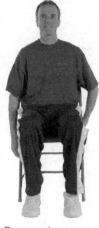

PHOTO 1

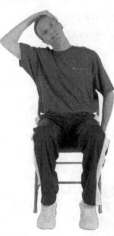

PHOTO 2

1. Sit up straight in a supportive, armless chair. Tighten your stomach muscles and tuck in your chin. Hold the underside of the chair with your left hand (photo 1).

2. Without moving your shoulders, tilt your head to the right so that your right earlobe moves toward your right shoulder.

3. Gently rest your right hand above your left ear (photo 2).

4. Hold this position for 30 to 60 seconds as you breathe deeply.

5. Return to the starting position.

6. Repeat this movement on the left.

7. Repeat this exercise 1 to 3 times on each side, alternating sides.

8. Perform this exercise once or twice a day.

Note: Once your neck muscles are loose, you can use a variation of this exercise to stretch the side of your trunk. Remove your hand from the underside of the chair, lean your body to the side, and gently stretch your head toward your hip.

#2 ■ Neck/Trunk Flexions and Hip Flexions/Abductions/ External Rotations

Why this exercise? This exercise will loosen the muscles, ligaments, and joints of the back of your neck, spine, and hips, which can tighten when you stay in 1 position for a long time.

1. Sit on the floor with your legs comfortably crossed in front of you. Tighten your stomach muscles and tuck in your chin (photo 1).

2. Clasp your hands behind your head, tilt your chin to your chest, and let the weight of your hands gently push your head down. Curl down as far as comfortably possible (photo 2).

3. Hold this position for 30 to 60 seconds as you breathe deeply.

4. Return to the starting position.

5. Repeat this movement 1 to 3 times.

6. Perform this exercise once or twice a day.

Note: If you have osteopenia (a significant decrease in bone density) or rounding or humping of your upper spine, do not do this exercise.

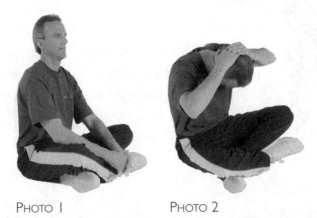

PHOTO 1   PHOTO 2

#3 ■ "W" Wall Stretches

Why this exercise? This exercise will loosen your shoulder muscles, ligaments, and joints, and will keep your back and neck straight and well aligned. It will make it easier to reach for an object on a high shelf.

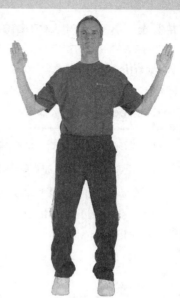

PHOTO 1

1. Stand with your back against a wall and your feet 18 to 24 inches from the wall and 6 to 8 inches apart. Tighten your stomach muscles and tuck in your chin.

2. Place your arms in a "W" position against the wall (photo 1).

3. Slide your arms up the wall as high as possible, making sure they stay flat against the wall as you lengthen your spine (photo 2).

4. Hold this position for 30 to 60 seconds as you breathe deeply.

5. Return to the starting position.

6. Repeat this movement 1 to 3 times.

7. Perform this exercise once or twice a day.

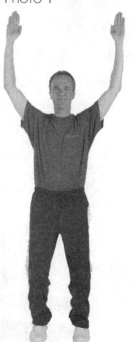

PHOTO 2

#4 ■ Shoulder Combined Movements

Why this exercise? This exercise will loosen your shoulder muscles, ligaments, and joints. It will make it easier to reach up to unscrew a light bulb or reach behind into your back pocket.

1. Sit up straight in a supportive chair. Do not lean back against the backrest. Tighten your stomach muscles and tuck in your chin.

2. Move your right hand, palm facing your back, up and over your right shoulder as far down your back as comfortably possible. Move your left hand, palm facing out, behind and up your back (photo 1).

3. Hold this position for 30 to 60 seconds as you breathe deeply (photo 2).

4. Return to the starting position.

5. Repeat this exercise by reversing the positions of your arms.

6. Repeat this movement 1 to 3 times on each side, alternating sides.

7. Perform this exercise once or twice a day.

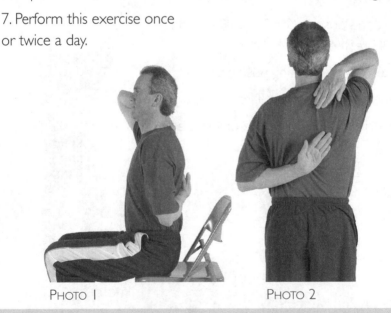

PHOTO 1   PHOTO 2

#5 ■ Spine Flexions/Hip Flexions and Extensions

Why this exercise? This exercise is great for stretching your front hip muscles, which may be tight from sitting too much. It will also loosen your spine, ligaments, and joints and will help you stand straighter and walk with a longer stride. Several of our clients have reported that they felt 2 inches taller after doing this exercise. That's because it opens tightened hips.

1. Lie on your back with your knees bent and your feet flat on the floor (photo 1). Tighten your stomach muscles and tuck in your chin.

2. Wrap your hands under your right thigh and pull your right knee as close as possible to your chest.

3. Straighten your left leg so that it is flat against the floor (photo 2).

4. Hold this position for 30 to 60 seconds as you breathe deeply.

5. Return to the starting position.

6. Repeat this exercise by reversing the positions of your legs.

7. Repeat this movement 1 to 3 times on each side, alternating sides.

8. Perform this exercise once or twice a day.

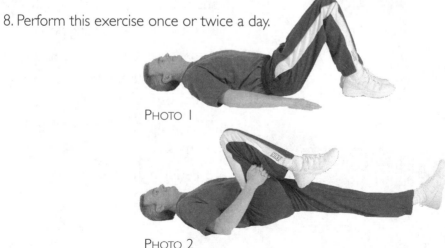

PHOTO 1

PHOTO 2

#6 ■ Spine and Neck Rotations

Why this exercise? This exercise will loosen your spine, neck muscles, ligaments, and joints—all of which can be tight as a result of inactivity. It will help you turn your spine more easily, which is necessary in golf, in tennis, and in backing your car out of the garage.

1. Lie on your back. Bend your knees, keeping your legs together and your feet close to your buttocks. Tighten your stomach muscles and tuck in your chin. Straighten your arms and stretch them out flat against the floor at shoulder height with your palms facing down (photo 1).

2. Lower your legs to the right, keeping them together and your knees bent (photo 2).

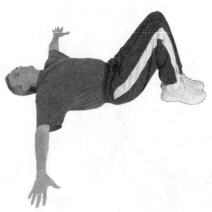

PHOTO 1

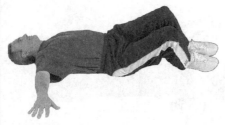

PHOTO 2

3. Keeping your shoulders flat on the floor, turn your head to the left.

4. Hold this position for 30 to 60 seconds as you breathe deeply.

5. Return to the starting position.

6. Repeat this exercise by dropping your knees to the left and turning your head to the right.

7. Repeat this movement 1 to 3 times.

8. Perform this exercise once or twice a day.

#7 ■ Spine Extensions

Why this exercise? This exercise loosens the muscles, ligaments, and joints of your spine, neck, and hands, which may be tight if you work at a computer. It will help you sit and stand straighter and will enhance the movement of your spine when you walk. **Caution:** If you feel any pain in your lower back when you do this exercise, stop. Do not do it again until you have consulted your physical therapist or physician.

1. Lie on your stomach on the floor. Tighten your stomach muscles and tuck in your chin.

2. Bend your elbows and keep your arms and hands flat on the floor with your fingers spread (photo 1).

3. Raise your head and upper body off the floor, keeping your arms on the floor and your fingers spread. Look straight ahead (photo 2).

4. Hold this position for 30 to 60 seconds as you breathe deeply.

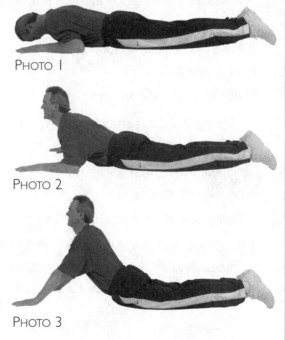

PHOTO 1

5. Return to the starting position.

6. Repeat this movement 1 to 3 times.

PHOTO 2

7. Perform this exercise once or twice a day.

Note: To increase the difficulty of this exercise, straighten and extend your arms while you raise your head and upper body (photo 3).

PHOTO 3

#8 ■ Leg Stretches

Why this exercise? This exercise will loosen your ligaments, joints, hamstrings, calves, and the muscles in your lower back. It will make it easier for you to bend and reach for objects and will help you avoid hamstring pulls.

1. Stand up straight. Move your right leg forward, keeping the heel on the floor. Put your weight on your left leg, bending the knee slightly. Place your hands on your left thigh. Tighten your stomach muscles and tuck in your chin (photo 1).

2. Lean forward, pushing your buttocks backward and keeping your back as straight as possible.

3. Reach for the toes of your right foot with your right hand (photo 2).

4. Hold this position for 30 to 60 seconds as you breathe deeply.

5. Return to the starting position.

6. Repeat this exercise by reversing the positions of your legs.

7. Repeat this movement 1 to 3 times on each side, alternating sides.

8. Perform this exercise once or twice a day.

Note: If you find this exercise uncomfortable or precarious, try the alternate hamstring stretch in chapter 2 (exercise 3, pages 46–47.)

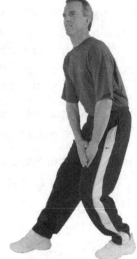

Photo 1

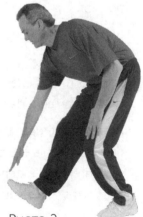

Photo 2

DAILY TIPS AND ENERGIZING IDEAS

This section includes easy-to-do tasks, modifications to daily routine, and hints to enhance and reinforce the exercises in your flexibility regimen. Place little notes to yourself everywhere you tend to look during the day as reminders to do them from time to time.

AT HOME AND WORK

■ When you finish bathing, your muscles are warm. That's a good time to stretch.

■ Do neck stretches while you watch television, sit at your desk, or stop at a traffic light.

■ Don't sit in the same position for too long—preferably not more than 30 minutes at a time.

■ Loosen your spine while you are sitting. Lean forward and down, reaching your hands to the floor. Then sit back up and gently arch your back.

■ While you are sitting, move your body away from the backrest of your chair, place your arms across your chest, and gently twist your trunk and neck to the right and left.

■ While you are standing in an elevator or waiting near a convenient wall, do the "W" stretch. This stretch also provides a nice break while you watch TV.

■ When you are driving long distances, get out of the car every 45 minutes to walk and do at least 1 stretch. If you are flying, walk up and down the aisle and do 1 or more stretches every 30 to 45 minutes.

IN THE GYM

■ Stretching before you exercise is not as effective as stretching afterward. Begin your exercise by warming up (such as walking for 5 minutes) and end with stretching.

■ If you don't want to stretch immediately after you have finished working out, spend a few minutes in a warm whirlpool bath or shower, then stretch.

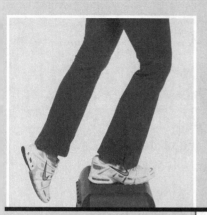

Chapter 6

■ ■ ■ ■ ■

Endurance

THE RIGHT SHOES

Workout shoes require extra shock absorption and protection, unlike those for everyday. Use the following list to select the right shoes:

■ The soles should be composed of shock-absorbing material. When you push on the sole, you should feel some give. The shoe should bend at the ball of your foot rather than in the middle.

■ The insole should mold to the shape of your foot. If you have a higher arch, the insoles should accommodate it. If your arch is flat, the insole should provide greater support.

■ The heel should always be low and compressible so it will absorb a lot of shock.

■ The material should let your foot breathe; shoes with some open weave on the top are best. The shoe should also lace through eyelets for added support.

■ The toe box should allow enough room for you to comfortably wiggle your toes.

■ The shoe should hold your heel firmly in place.

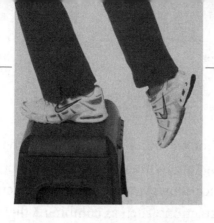

*You have to run faster and faster
just to stay in the same place!*

—THE RED QUEEN IN *THROUGH THE
LOOKING-GLASS* BY LEWIS CARROLL

Endurance is a combination of aerobic capacity, cardiopulmonary performance, and stamina. Whether you are running a marathon, walking the dog, or learning to use a new walker—and whether you're 29, 59, or 89—endurance enables you to do what you want to do for as long as you want to do it. The bad news is that as you age, you must work harder to maintain your level of fitness. The good news is that you can improve your capacity every day. Raising your endurance levels will provide you with the stamina and vitality you need to develop your posture, strength, balance, and flexibility.

Phil, 52, was quite an athlete in high school. The first time he came up to bat in his law firm's softball game, he hit one out of the park. That crack of the bat felt great! He didn't feel so great, however, after running the bases. He couldn't believe how out of breath he was when he crossed home plate.

PROPER ENDURANCE

Endurance is the body's ability to sustain an activity over a period of time. There are 2 basic types: muscular and cardiovascular.

Muscular endurance allows you to perform any activity that requires repeated muscle contractions, such as climbing 3 flights of stairs. It is best achieved through strength training with increased numbers of repetitions, such as the exercises in chapter 3.

Cardiovascular endurance allows you to walk, run, jump rope, swim, or perform any other activity that uses large body muscles (such as those in the front of the thigh and the buttocks) over a prolonged period of time. Healthy cardiovascular endurance enables your lungs, heart, and circulatory system to function efficiently so that you don't develop shortness of breath or excessive fatigue.

Some activities require both cardiovascular and muscular endurance. Your lungs, heart, and circulatory system must function efficiently to comfortably climb 3 flights of stairs, but so must your leg muscles.

If you have any coronary artery disease risk factors (Chart 1, page 227), we recommend that you seek the guidance of your physician before you start any conditioning program.

This chapter focuses on improving your cardiovascular endurance. To accomplish this, you need to know how to check your heart rate, and then how to set your target heart rate.

CHECKING YOUR HEART RATE

This is the most accurate way to check your resting heart rate: On 4 consecutive mornings, before you get out of bed, count the number of times your heart beats in 1 full minute. The best way to do this is to take your radial pulse at your wrist artery. Place your right index and middle fingers against the inside of your left wrist just below the base of your thumb

Chart I

RISK FACTORS FOR CORONARY ARTERY DISEASE

Modifiable Risk Factors (Those you can control)	Non-Modifiable Risk Factors (Those you cannot control)
High blood pressure	Age (men over age 45, women over age 55)
High cholesterol levels	Race (whites have a greater risk)
Good cholesterol/bad cholesterol ratio	Gender (men are at higher risk until age 70
High triglyceride levels	when risk evens out)
Smoking	Family history of heart disease
Second-hand smoke	Fibrinogen levels in blood
Obesity	Enlargement of left ventricle
High stress level	Previous heart attack
Sedentary lifestyle	History of heart valve or peripheral
High blood sugar levels/Diabetes	vascular problems
Diet	
Poor education about heart health	

(photo 1). Press gently; if you press too firmly you might not get an accurate reading. After recording your resting heart rate for 4 consecutive mornings, calculate the average of the 4 readings. A resting heart rate is usually between 60 to 80 beats per minute (BPM), although a rate of 60 to 100 beats per minute is considered normal.

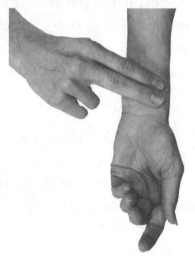

Once you are proficient at finding and counting your pulse, you can use a shortcut. Count your heart rate for 10 seconds and multiply the number by 6. This gives you your heart rate for 1 minute.

PHOTO I

Before you begin exercising, relax in a chair for 1 minute, and then take your resting heart rate. You are now ready to monitor your heart rate while exercising aerobically.

To see how activity affects your heart rate, take your resting heart rate and then jump or run in place for 2 minutes. Take your pulse immediately afterward. Depending on your aerobic condition, your pulse should rise anywhere from a few beats to more than 20 beats per minute. Continue to exercise for the next 10 minutes, taking your pulse every 2 minutes. Your heart rate should return to its resting level 2 to 20 minutes after you've finished the exercise.

You should check your pulse before, during, and after any endurance exercise. Keep a log and record your heart rate at least once a week; you should be able not only to see an improvement in your heart's ability to recover, but also to chart the increase in your aerobic capacity, or cardiovascular endurance.

DETERMINING YOUR TARGET OR EXERCISE HEART RATE

Before starting an exercise program, you will need to know your resting heart rate (RHR), your maximum heart rate (MHR), and your target heart rate (THR). Your target heart rate is the goal you should strive to reach when you are exercising. It is calculated using the following formula:

THR = RHR + 55% to 85% (MHR – RHR)

The formula looks complicated, but it is relatively simple to follow with a little guidance.

1) Determine your resting heart rate (RHR) by taking your pulse in the morning before you get out of bed (See pages 226-227).

2) Determine your maximum heart rate (MHR) by subtracting your age from 220.

3) Subtract your RHR from your MHR.

4) Establish the level of intensity at which your exercise will be most effective. This number is expressed as a percentage, ranging from 55 to 85 percent, depending on your physical condition. If you are out of shape, then 55 percent may be a reasonable target. If you have been inactive for a long period, you might even use a lower percentage. If you already exercise regularly, 70 percent may be a better target. Work toward a goal of 80 to 85 percent as your condition improves.

5) Multiply the level of intensity percentage by the number you got when you subtracted your RHR from your MHR.

6) The final number is your target heart rate (THR).

It is difficult to keep your heart rate at the same level during aerobic exercise, so you can use plus or minus 10 percent of your target heart rate as your THR range.

The following example might help clarify the formula. An out-of-shape 50-year-old woman with a RHR of 80 beats per minute decides that she should exercise at 55 percent of her MHR. This is how she determines her THR:

$$80 + 55\% (220 - 50 - 80) = 130$$
$$130 + 10\% = 143$$
$$130 - 10\% = 117$$

This 50-year-old's THR would be 130 beats per minute (BPM). During aerobic exercise, she would strive to keep her heart rate between 117 and 143 BPM.

A 60-year-old man with a resting heart rate of 68 BPM has been on a power walk program of 3 miles per day 4 times a week. His goal is to exercise at 80 percent of his MHR. He would determine his target heart rate as follows:

$$68 + 80\% (220 - 60 - 68) = 142$$
$$142 + 10\% = 156$$
$$142 - 10\% = 128$$

His THR would be 142 beats per minute. During aerobic exercise, he would strive to keep his heart rate between 128 and 156 BPM.

To improve your endurance, you should exercise at 60 to 85 percent of your maximum heart rate, but you may need to work up to that level.

We strongly advise you to calculate your target heart rate using the method we described, but for a quick estimate, you can use Chart 2 as a guide. This chart shows average heart rate ranges based on the age of normal, healthy individuals without any risk of coronary artery disease. (You are at a higher risk if you have a family history of coronary artery disease, diabetes, high cholesterol and triglyceride levels, high blood pressure, or obesity. You may also be at risk if you do not participate in regular aerobic exercise, if you are a smoker, or if you experience high stress levels)

Chart 2

HEART RATE RANGES
DURING EXERCISE

Age	Desired Range for Heart Rate During Exercise
40	126–153
50	119–145
60	112–136
70	105–128
80	98–119
90	91–111
100	84–102

Caution: If you take medication that alters your heart rate or blood pressure (such as vasodilators, calcium channel blockers, angiotensin-converting enzyme inhibitor, and alpha and beta-adrenergic blockers), or if you have a pacemaker, an irregular heart rhythm (atrial fibrillation), or any other condition that affects your pulse rate, do not use the target heart rate method to make decisions about your endurance training. Your heart rate is a reflection of how hard your body works. Because these medications and conditions can slow your heart rate, you might not be able to reach the heart rate derived from the target heart rate calculation; if you try to do so, you may end up overexerting yourself.

ENDURANCE CHANGES

Your cardiopulmonary capacity is significantly reduced as a result of a combination of age-related changes and little or no exercise. Starting in the mid-twenties, cardiovascular system fitness declines by about 8 percent per decade for inactive adults and about 4 percent per decade for physically active adults. As you age, your maximum heart rate declines. Your heart's ability to pump blood and use oxygen efficiently is lower both when you are at rest and when you exercise, and your blood pressure at rest is higher.

The loss of elasticity in the aorta (the large artery that carries blood from the heart), leads to a 1 percent decrease in the output of the heart each year. A loss of elasticity may also occur in the peripheral arteries and veins. Varicose veins and a rise in blood pressure (at the rate of about 1 percent per year) may develop as a result of these changes. Degenerative changes in heart valves may also contribute to high blood pressure, irregular heart rhythms, a decrease in maximum heart rate, and sometimes the presence of heart murmurs.

As you age, you may develop orthostatic hypotension (see page 157), a drop in blood pressure that occurs when you move from lying to sitting or sitting to standing. This can lead to dizziness or light-headedness.

The pulmonary system also undergoes changes related to aging. Lung tissue stiffens and loses elasticity; as a result, your lungs operate less effectively, requiring you to breathe more frequently. You may become more susceptible to respiratory problems. Chapter 2 discusses spinal degeneration leading to a loss of height, rounding of the upper back, and a loss of rib cage flexibility. These changes also can make breathing less efficient and may cause shortness of breath. If you combine these age-related changes with a lifetime of little or no exercise, you will experience a significant reduction in lung capacity.

ANATOMICAL AND HEALTH INFORMATION

Cardiovascular/Pulmonary Systems

Thoracic Cavity

The thoracic cavity or thorax is the bone and cartilage framework that houses and protects the heart, lungs, and major vessels of the vascular system (Figure 6.1). The thorax is composed of 12 pairs of ribs, the sternum or breastbone, and 12 thoracic vertebrae.

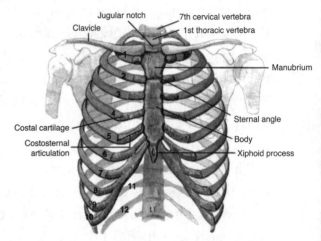

FIGURE 6.1

Circulatory System

The circulatory or vascular system is composed of the heart, blood vessels, and lymph vessels. This system brings oxygen, hormones, chemicals, nutrients, and antibodies to all body tissues and eliminates carbon dioxide and other waste products.

Heart

The heart is a hollow muscular organ shaped like a blunt cone and about the size of your fist (Figure 6.2). It is located behind the breastbone. It is a simple pump, or more accurately, a pair of pumps that beat between 60 and 100 times per

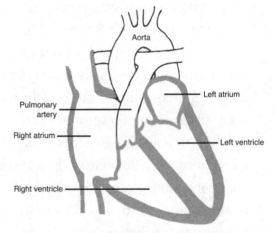

FIGURE 6.2

minute. The heart is divided into 4 chambers—2 upper chambers called atria that receive blood into the heart, and 2 lower chambers called ventricles that pump blood away from the heart to the lungs and to the rest of the body. The pericardium is a fluid membranous sac that surrounds the heart and provides a frictionless environment.

Blood Vessels

Blood vessels are divided into 3 main groups: arteries, veins, and capillaries. The right and left coronary arteries (Figure 6.3) supply blood to the heart walls. These arteries arise from the aorta, encircle the outside of the heart, divide into several branches, and provide circulation to many overlapping areas of the heart. The overlap serves as safety factors in the case of a blocked artery or heart attack.

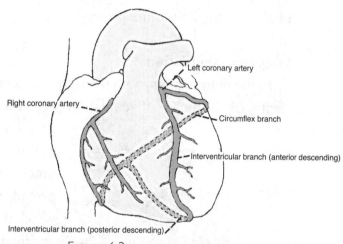

FIGURE 6.3

The rest of your arteries carry oxygenated blood to your head, neck, arms, legs, and all of your inner organs. Blood leaves your heart via the aorta, then enters other arteries that decrease in size and eventually branch off into small arterioles and even smaller capillaries. The capillaries provide all body cells with nutrients and oxygen and pick up waste products including carbon dioxide. Capillaries also become veins, which carry the blood (with its carbon dioxide and other waste products) to body organs such as the liver and kidneys for cleansing and then to the heart and back to the lungs for reoxygenation.

Lymph Vessels

Lymph vessels form a network in the body and are responsible for conveying tissue-cleaning fluid from the tissues to the bloodstream. The fluid is similar to blood but does not contain red blood cells. Its primiary responsibility is to carry nutrients to the cells of the body and collect waste products. When the fluid is returned to the bloodstream by the lymphatic system, it becomes plasma.

Lungs and Ventilation

In the pulmonary system the right and left lungs, located in the chest cavity, are the organs of ventilation (Figure 6.4). The pleura (a membranous sac filled with a small amount of fluid) cover each lung and line the inner part of the thoracic cage to provide a frictionless environment in which the lungs inflate and deflate approximately 12 to 20 times per minute. Oxygen-rich air is taken in either through the nose or mouth and travels through the pharynx (the tube that goes as far as the Adam's apple); the larynx, which contains the vocal cords (a continuation of the tube); the trachea; the bronchi; and finally into each lung. Once in the lungs, the bronchi grow smaller, branching into bronchioles and finally alveoli. It is at the alveolar level that gas exchange (taking in oxygen and giving off carbon dioxide) actually occurs.

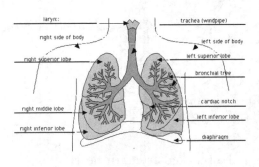

FIGURE 6.4

Muscle contraction enables air to be brought into the lungs, and muscle relaxation allows air to flow back out of the lungs. The primary muscle responsible for bringing air into the lungs is the diaphragm, a large dome-shaped muscle separating the thoracic cavity from the abdominal cavity. The intercostals—the muscles between the ribs—also help bring air into the lungs. Forced exhalation in the form of a cough or sneeze is usually the result of abdominal muscle action.

Health-related Conditions

Endurance is affected by age, but also by some health-related conditions, such as coronary artery disease, peripheral vascular disease, and chronic obstructive pulmonary disease. Each reduces the body's ability to provide the blood and oxygen needed for aerobic activities. If you have any of these conditions, please contact your physician before beginning an exercise program. After appropriate treatment, starting or returning to a program of increasing physical activity will enhance your fitness and functional ability.

Coronary Artery Disease

Coronary artery disease (CAD) is a condition in which the heart muscle receives an inadequate amount of oxygen due to a blockage of the coronary blood supply. The most common causes are atherosclerosis (an accumulation of fatty substances in the linings of the arteries) and coronary artery spasm (a sudden contraction of coronary artery muscles that causes the vessel to narrow). The symptoms of CAD may range from angina (mild chest pain) to myocardial infarction (a heart attack). Myocardial infarction may range from mild to severe, depending on the damage to the heart wall muscle.

There are many risk factors for CAD; some you can control and some you cannot. You can have some effect on high blood pressure, high cholesterol and triglyceride levels, smoking, obesity, high stress levels, sedentary lifestyle, and diabetes. You can't do anything about your age

(CAD often affects persons over age 40), race (it is most common in Caucasians), gender (it is a greater risk for males until age 70, when the risk for men and women evens out), and other inherited factors.

Prevention is the first line of defense against CAD; you should work to improve or eliminate all of the factors that are within your control. Treatment may include medication, conditioning exercises, endurance training, stress management, diet modification, smoking cessation, angioplasty (surgery to open the blocked artery), and coronary artery bypass grafting surgery.

Peripheral Vascular Disease

Peripheral vascular disease occurs when there is a blockage of or decrease in the blood flow through either the arteries or the veins in the arms or legs. If the disease affects the arteries, it may eventually lead to tissue death. Arterial circulation difficulty is characterized by muscle cramps, particularly in the calves, that occur during walking or exercise and are eased by rest. If the disease affects the veins, it may lead to the development of varicose veins, leg swelling, and ulcers.

Chronic Obstructive Pulmonary Diseases

Chronic obstructive pulmonary diseases (COPD) include asthma, bronchiectasis, chronic bronchitis, cystic fibrosis, and emphysema. These diseases may result in breathing difficulty, chronic cough, excessive mucus production, wheezing, and shortness of breath.

Asthma affects both children and adults. Severe blocking of the airways may occur as a result of a spasm of the air passages, increased accumulation of mucus in the airways, or swelling of the airways. Asthma may be caused by allergic reactions, lung infections, emotional stress, drug reactions, irritation of the lung tubes, and certain climate conditions. Exercise-induced asthma can occur after short spurts (6 to 8 minutes) of intense physical activity.

Bronchiectasis is a chronic condition in which the bronchi abnormally stretch and may become irregularly shaped. The disease is usually associated with inflamed airways, infections in the bronchi, and obstructions of the airways. It may occur following a lung infection or when foreign substances become lodged in the bronchi.

Chronic bronchitis is associated with persistent irritation of the bronchi (large passageways in the lungs), leading to obstruction of the airways. Chronic bronchitis is often associated with environmental and occupational pollutants, cigarette smoking, and chronic infections. It may also be hereditary.

Cystic fibrosis is an inherited disease characterized by accumulations of very thick mucus in the lungs, as well as abnormal secretions of saliva and sweat.

Emphysema is a chronic lung disease characterized by overinflation of the alveoli (the small sacs of the lungs) and may be associated with excessive mucus production. It occurs more often in men than women, may be hereditary, and is frequently found in heavy smokers. Individuals with emphysema often exhibit shortness of breath, a barrel-shaped chest, an increased use of neck muscles to assist inhalation, pursed lips used to blow out air to facilitate breathing, and an increased rounding of the upper and mid back.

Treatment programs for patients with COPD may include breathing and conditioning exercises, lung clearing techniques, endurance training, relaxation and energy conservation techniques, prevention of pulmonary infections, appropriate nutrition, and respiratory muscle strength training.

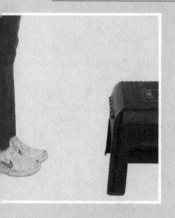
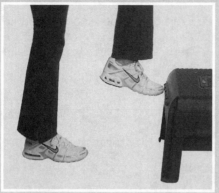
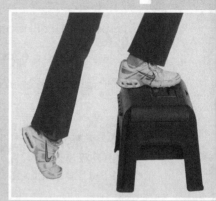

ENDURANCE ASSESSMENT

This section contains 3 tests: 2 to assess your endurance capabilities and 1 to assess your breathing capabilities. You only need to take 1 of the endurance assessments; you may choose which.

Take your resting heart rate right before you begin your endurance test. After you have completed the test, make sure that your heart rate has returned to the resting rate before you begin another assessment or exercise. We recommend that you take your heart rate at 2 minutes and 10 minutes after finishing.

Caution: If you have had any past cardiac or respiratory problems, consult your physician before you take these tests.

Your heart rate and the Borg Scale of Perceived Exertion (see next page) will be your guides for how much aerobic conditioning activity you can and should do.

The Borg Scale of Perceived Exertion was developed by Gunnar Borg, PhD, and is the primary method used to measure exertion. Use the scale (Chart 3) to determine how hard you are exercising.

Chart 3

BORG SCALE OF
PERCEIVED EXERTION

Least Effort

6		
7	very, very light	
8		
9	very light	
10		
11	fairly light	
12		*Endurance*
13	somewhat hard	*Training*
14		*Zone*
15	hard	
16		*Strength*
17	very hard	*Training*
		Zone
18		
19	very, very hard	
20		

Maximum Effort

Look at the words and numbers on the right side of the scale. For example, while reading this text, your effort should be "very, very light" or a score of 6 or 7 (the number next to the words). If you were to run up and down all the bleachers at a football stadium, you might choose "very, very hard" or a score of 19. According to Borg, the numbers are approximately related to your actual heart rate during various levels of exertion; multiply the number on the scale by 10 to arrive at an approximate heart rate. In the above examples, the score of 7 would equate to an approximate heart rate of 70, and the score of 19 to a heart rate of 190. For testing purposes, gradually work your way up to 13 or "somewhat hard." **Caution:** If you experience chest pain, shortness of breath, dizziness, weakness, or clamminess, stop exercising and consult your physician.

ROCKPORT WALKING TEST

Before performing this test, you must identify a route of exactly 1 mile. It can be inside or outside. Shopping malls and walking trails often have the mileage marked.

Action: Before beginning the test, take your resting heart rate (pages 226-228). Record your RHR and the time you begin. Walk a mile as fast as you can.

Score: At the end of the mile, record your time. Take your heart rate immediately and record it.

Time: _____ Time: _____ Time: _____

RHR: _____ RHR: _____ RHR: _____

Final HR: _____ Final HR: _____ Final HR: _____

Date: _____ Date: _____ Date: _____

Chart 4			**Chart 5**		
NORMS FOR MEN FOR THE ROCKPORT WALKING TEST			NORMS FOR WOMEN FOR THE ROCKPORT WALKING TEST		
Age 40-49	High	100–200 HR in 9 to 15 min.	Age 40-49	High	100–200 HR in 10 to 15 min.
	Avg	100–200 HR in 18 to 21 min.		Avg	100–200 HR in 17.5 to 19.5 min.
	Low	140–200 HR in over 22 min.		Low	130–200 HR in over 20 min.
Age 50-59	High	100–180 HR in 10 to 14 min.	Age 50-59	High	100–170 HR in 11 to 15.5 min.
	Avg	100–200 HR in 17 to 21 min.		Avg	100–200 HR in 17.5 to 19 min.
	Low	140–200 HR in over 22 min.		Low	100–200 HR in over 21 min.
Age 60 plus	High	100–175 HR in 10 to 14 min.	Age 60 plus	High	100–170 HR in 12 to 16 min.
	Avg	100–200 HR in 17 to 20 min.		Avg	100–200 HR in 18 to 20 min.
	Low	120–200 HR in over 22 min.		Low	100–200 HR in over 22 min.

Assessment: Compare your heart rate taken immediately after you completed the test with Charts 4 and 5. If you are below the average for your age and gender, select an activity from 8 Great Exercises for Endurance.

KASCH STEP TEST

This functional fitness test is based upon the principle that the better your fitness level, the sooner your heart rate will return to its pre-exercise level after exercising. You will need a 12-inch high step or sturdy bench, a stopwatch, and a metronome. Set the metronome at 96, which will provide a stepping rate of 24 steps per minute. If you do not have a metronome, create the correct rhythm by stepping as you count one thousand one, one thousand two, one thousand three, and so on.

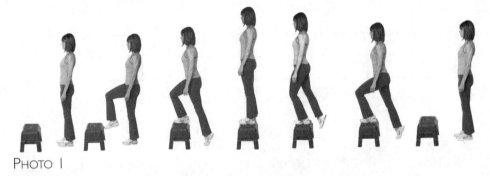

PHOTO 1

Action: Before beginning the test, take and record your resting heart rate. For 3 minutes, climb onto and off of the step, beginning with your right leg. Place your right leg completely onto the step, followed

Chart 6
SCORING METHOD FOR THE KASCH STEP TEST

Fitness Rating	MALES		FEMALES	
	RHR	Final HR	RHR	Final HR
Excellent	50–55	70–78	55–60	72–83
Good	56–62	79–90	61–65	84–97
Above Average	63–66	91–97	66–69	98–106
Average	67–70	98–105	70–73	107–117
Below Average	71–75	106–117	74–79	118–127
Poor	76–83	118–130	80–85	128–140
Very Poor	84–95	131–165	86–100	141–155

by your left leg. Then take your right leg off of the step completely, followed by your left leg. Alternate legs, so that you will then start with your left leg (photo 1).

Score: At the end of 3 minutes, immediately take and record your heart rate.

Resting HR:	Resting HR:	Resting HR:
Final HR:	Final HR:	Final HR:
Date:	Date:	Date:

Assessment: Compare your results with Chart 6. If your results were Below Average or worse, select an activity from 8 Great Exercises for Endurance.

15-COUNT SCALE

This is a simple breathing test.

Action: Use a stopwatch to time yourself as you breathe in deeply. Count to 15 as you exhale, and continue exhaling until you reach 15. It should take you 8 seconds or less to exhale and count to 15.

Score: Record the time it took you to complete this test.

| Score: | Score: | Score: |
| Date: | Date: | Date: |

Assessment: If you needed 2 breaths or it took longer you than 8 seconds to exhale and count to 15, consult your physician or physical therapist before starting an endurance program.

Wendy's Prescription for Endurance

Wendy was shocked to find that she was below the norms for her age on the Kasch Step Test. She decided it was time to improve her endurance and started walking for 45 minutes, 5 days a week.

James's Prescription for Endurance

James scored in the low range on the Rockport Walking Test. He decided to ride an indoor recumbent bicycle for 20 minutes, 4 times a week.

PRESCRIPTION FOR ENDURANCE

Date:_____

Rockport Walking Test

Time: _____

RHR: _____

Final HR: _____

Exercise(s) Needed: _____

Kasch Step Test

RHR: _____

Final HR: _____

Exercise(s) Needed: _____

15-Count Scale

Time: _____

(Make a copy for your personal use)

8 GREAT EXERCISES FOR ENDURANCE

#1 Walking

#2 Cycling

#3 Jumping Rope

#4 Water Jogging and Aerobics

#5 Stepping

#6 Skiing

#7 Rowing

#8 Circuit Program

Note: Other chapters assign 1 or more of 8 exercises based on the results of your assessment. In this chapter, we recommend 8 different kinds of aerobic endurance activities; you may choose 1 or any combination you prefer.

Once your program is in place, you can exercise anywhere—indoors, outdoors, at home, on the road, at a fitness club, or at a community center. The key to success is finding the environment and activities that best meet your needs.

Endurance activities have many benefits:

■ **Health benefits.** Over time, aerobic conditioning will improve the performance of your heart, circulation, and lungs, and will reduce your risk of coronary heart disease.

■ **Weight loss.** Many studies support the use of endurance exercise along with an appropriate diet, to lose or control weight. Exercise alone can help you lose weight. We have many clients who never exercised before; when they started an endurance program, their weight decreased though their calorie intake did not. Combining proper exercise with a healthy diet, however, produces even more impressive results. **Note:** Exercising may make you hungry. For the greatest benefit, make a special effort to control your eating while continuing your exercise program.

When planning your endurance activities, consider these 5 factors:

■ **Intensity:** Exercise at an appropriate level of difficulty. Work toward a goal of 70 to 85 percent of your maximum heart rate and a rate of perceived exertion that is "somewhat hard" to "hard."

■ **Frequency:** Exercise 3 to 5 times per week for the best results.

- **Duration:** Make each exercise session last between 30 and 60 minutes.

- **Mode:** Select any type of exercise that uses your large body muscles (especially those in the lower legs—the buttocks, the front thigh muscles, and the back calf muscles). You can work out indoors or outdoors and with or without equipment.

- **Dosage:** Exercise continuously or try interval training, which inserts rest times between various activities.

How much effort?

- It doesn't take much effort to talk during moderate activity, but it can be difficult during vigorous activity. If you can't talk while you're exercising, you're working too hard. If you can sing a song, you're not working hard enough.

- You should not perspire during light activity unless the weather is hot. You will—and should—perspire during vigorous or sustained moderate activity, regardless of the temperature.

- Your muscles will feel fine after moderate activity, but they may feel rubbery after vigorous activity. If your muscles are overtired after your exercise session, cut back to a lower level of activity and work your way back up gradually.

Indoors or out?

- If you exercise outdoors, the varied environment will keep you fresh and interested, but inclement weather can sometimes make exercising unpleasant.

- If you exercise indoors, you can control the climate, but you can easily become bored.

- Vary your routine by including both indoor and outdoor activities.

How To Create an Endurance Routine

1. Begin any endurance training program with a warm-up period. Gradually increase the intensity of your activity over a period of 5 to 10 minutes.

2. Start with a comfortable pace, speed, and distance. Start slowly and gradually increase your pace and intensity. As your fitness improves, you will need to work harder to achieve your target heart rate. Increase your speed and/or intensity—choose a route with more hills or increase the elevation and/or resistance on the machine.

3. Keep your heart rate in your target range for at least 20 minutes, unless you are jumping rope (in which case 5 to 10 minutes may be strenuous enough) or following a circuit program (special instructions for this type of program are given later in this chapter). Maintain your target heart rate as much as possible after you warm up and until you cool down.

4. End your workout with a 5- to 10-minute cool-down period. Gradually reduce the intensity of your activity so that your heart can return to pre-exercise levels.

Caution: Always listen to your body and be alert to any signs and symptoms of too much stress.

#1 ■ Walking

Why this exercise? Our definition of walking can include jogging, running, and skating, depending on your level of physical fitness. Most of these variations can be performed outdoors or indoors. Walking is a weight-bearing exercise, which is good for bone density, but it may irritate your joints, especially those in your knees, hips, and ankles.

Outdoors

Getting out into the fresh air and conquering the roads and hills— at whatever pace you can achieve—is the ideal way to begin an aerobic exercise program. You can begin by walking out your front door.

Pros

- You can walk almost anywhere.
- You don't need much, if any, equipment.
- You can walk with friends.
- You can listen to music or recorded books while exercising.

Cons

- The weather can be a problem.
- You're dependent on your body for feedback on your performance, unless you use a heart monitor.

Indoors

You can walk indoors using a treadmill or an elliptical machine. Your imagination can take you along the Appalachian Trail or a Cape Cod beach, through a Central American cloud forest, or to a pueblo ruin in the Southwest.

Pros

■ The weather is not a problem.

■ You can adjust the equipment for grade and speed.

■ Machines provide feedback on your speed, calories burned, miles covered, incline, and elapsed time.

■ You can watch TV, listen to music or recorded books, or read while you exercise.

Cons

■ You need equipment and a place to use it.

■ Using the same machine in the same location may become boring.

Tips for walking:

■ Walk with your head and back well aligned and your stomach and chin tucked in. Your toes should point forward, your shoulders should be down and relaxed, and your arms should be close to your body. Keep your elbows bent 90 degrees and let your arms swing comfortably, but not higher than the middle of your chest and not past your hips in the back. As you increase your pace of walking, you will increase the movement of the arms as well. You hands should be relaxed and in a loose fist. As you take a step, put your weight on your heel and then roll toward the front of your foot to push off.

■ Time, not distance, is important. Gradually increase the time you walk to 30 to 60 minutes.

■ To enhance your workout, try not to hold onto the handrails of the treadmill or elliptical while you use them. If you must do so, use a very light grip.

■ Pay attention to your body! If you experience pain, seek professional assistance before you hurt yourself.

#2 ■ Cycling

Why this exercise? You can cycle outdoors or indoors. Bicycling is less weight-bearing than walking, jogging, running, and skating, so it may put less stress on your lower body, but it may irritate your joints, especially your knees. Recumbent bicycles and cycle ergometers are the least stressful options.

Outdoors

You can bicycle outdoors in the fresh air, traversing the roads at your own pace.

Pros

■ You can bike almost anywhere.

■ You can bicycle with friends.

■ You can listen to music or recorded books while exercising.

Cons

■ The weather can be a problem.

■ You're dependent on your body for feedback on your performance, unless you use a heart rate monitor.

Indoors

You can bicycle indoors using stationary or recumbent bicycles, or cycle ergometers. If you have painful knees, spinal stenosis, or spondylolisthesis (when a vertabrae slips in front of the one below it), a recumbent bicycle is a better choice.

Pros

■ The weather is not a problem.

■ You can adjust the equipment for grade and speed.

■ Machines provide feedback on your speed, calories burned, miles covered, and elapsed time.

- You can watch TV, listen to music or recorded books, or read while exercising.

Cons

- You need equipment and a place to use it.

- Using the same machine in the same location may become boring.

Tips for cycling:

- To ensure proper seat height on an upright or recumbent bicycle, place your feet on the pedals. Your knee should be almost fully extended—just slightly bent—when your leg is in the bottom position. If you use an arm cycling machine, adjust the seat height so that your nose is at the top-most portion of the arm crank.

- Time, not distance, is important. Gradually increase the time you bike to 30 to 60 minutes.

- Try aerobic cross-training; walk 1 day and cycle on another.

#3 ■ Jumping Rope

Why this exercise? This is a weight-bearing exercise that requires balance and coordination. Because it is a particularly strenuous activity, you can accomplish more in less time, but it may be stressful on your back and lower leg joints. Since a jump rope is portable it can be used in almost any environment, whether at home or on the road.

Pros

- You can jump rope almost anywhere, indoors or out.

- The weather is not a problem.

- You don't need much equipment and it's inexpensive.

- You can watch TV or listen to music or recorded books while you exercise.

Cons

■ You're dependent on your body for feedback on your performance, unless you use a heart rate monitor.

■ Jumping rope may irritate your joints, especially those in your hips, knees, ankles, or back.

■ It may challenge your balance and coordination.

■ It may become boring.

Tips for jumping rope:

■ To make sure that your jump rope is the right length, stand on the center of the rope with your feet shoulder-width apart; the handles should be about 2 inches above your hips.

■ You may jump rope using both feet at the same time or alternating feet.

■ Jumping rope is a very strenuous activity, so start with just 30 to 60 seconds. You can gradually increase your time until your heart rate is in the target range for 5 to 10 minutes (or more).

#4 ■ Water Jogging and Aerobics

Why this exercise? Exercising in a pool takes advantage of the physical properties of water that both assist and resist movement. Water exercise is very easy on your back and lower legs since gravity is not a factor. The effects on bone density depend on your activity. Water jogging is not weight-bearing. The weight-bearing force of water aerobics varies, based on how many activities like jumping are incorporated.

Pros

■ Water aerobics require little coordination and skill.

■ You can exercise with friends.

Cons

■ You're dependent on your body for feedback on your performance.

■ You have to have access to a pool.

■ Pool chemicals, such as chlorine, may irritate your skin and eyes.

Tips for water jogging and aerobics:

■ Time, not distance, is important.

■ Gradually increase the time you perform water jogging or aerobics to 30 to 60 minutes.

■ If you decide to try water jogging, be sure you obtain a well-fitting aqua jogging belt.

#5 ■ Stepping

Why this exercise? Stepping includes stairs and machines, such as mechanical steppers, steppers with revolving stairs, and climbers. Stepping is a weight-bearing exercise, which is good for your bone density, but it may irritate your joints, especially your knees, hips, and ankles. Stepping may also contribute to substantial increase in the strength of your lower leg extensor muscle (buttocks, anterior thighs, and posterior calf).

Pros

■ The weather is not a problem.

■ You can adjust the equipment for grade and speed.

■ Machines provide feedback on your speed, calories burned, steps climbed, incline, and elapsed time.

■ You can watch TV, listen to music or recorded books, or read while you exercise.

Cons

■ You need equipment and a place to use it.

■ Using the same equipment in the same location may become boring.

Tips for stepping:

■ Do not bounce when you step; your motion should be smooth.

■ Start slowly and gradually increase your pace and intensity.

■ Time is important. Gradually increase the time you step to 30 to 60 minutes.

■ To enhance your workout on steppers or revolving stairs, try not to hold onto the machine. If you must do so, use a very light grip.

■ Use your imagination to keep your workout interesting. Pretend you're climbing Mt. Everest when you use a stepper, especially during the first and last few minutes—the times that are always the most difficult.

#6 ■ Skiing

Why this exercise? You can ski cross-country outdoors or on a machine indoors. Skiing is a weight-bearing activity, which is good for bone density. It exercises both your arms and your legs, but it may irritate your joints, especially those in your knees, hips, and ankles.

Outdoors

Getting out in the mountain air and conquering the hills or cross-country trails—at whatever pace you can achieve—provides a beautiful environment in which to develop your endurance.

Pros

- Cross-country skiing is a great opportunity to get out during winter.
- You can ski with friends.
- You can listen to music or recorded books while exercising.

Cons

- The weather can be a problem.
- Joint pain may be exacerbated by the cold.
- You're dependent on your body for feedback on your performance, unless you use a heart rate monitor.

Indoors

You can ski indoors using a ski machine. Your imagination can take you to the Rockies or the Alps or to a quiet trail in New England.

Pros

- The weather is not a problem.
- You can adjust the equipment for grade and speed.

■ Machines provide feedback on your speed, calories burned, miles covered, incline, and elapsed time.

■ You can watch TV, listen to music or recorded books, or read while you exercise.

Cons

■ You need equipment and a place to use it.

■ Using the same machine in the same location may become boring.

Tips for skiing:

■ Time, not distance, is important. Gradually increase the time you ski to 30 to 60 minutes.

■ If you want to see if you would like skiing, loop the Thera-band® around a stable object at waist height; you can use a newel post or a support column in your basement. Hold the ends of the band in your hands and pull, alternating your arms.

#7 ■ Rowing

Why this exercise? Rowing exercises both your arms and legs and is partially weight-bearing, but will not be as hard on your joints as other activities. Because most people do not have easy access to a boat, the information in this section is limited to rowing machines.

Pros

■ The weather is not a problem.

■ You can adjust the equipment for resistance.

■ Machines provide feedback on your performance.

- You can watch TV or listen to music or recorded books while you exercise.

Cons

- You need equipment and a place to use it.

- Using the same machine in the same location may become boring.

Tips for rowing:

- Time is important. Gradually increase the time you row to 30 to 60 minutes.

- After you have successfully increased your time, you can then increase your speed and resistance.

- Imagine yourself with a rowing team pushing to beat the competition or picture yourself alone in the boat skimming gently through the water on a magnificent day.

#8 ■ Circuit Program

Why this exercise? Circuit aerobic training is done in a gym. You can incorporate any number of machines into your program, including treadmills, arm cycling machines, bicycles, rowing machines, elliptical machines, and climbers. Several of these activities are weight-bearing and will enhance bone density; some may be stressful on your back and lower leg joints. Circuit training exercises both your arms and legs.

An aerobic circuit program is great when you need a change and some variety, but it's not a good option for beginners. It can be confusing and it takes a while to learn the different machines and determine proper settings for each of them. If you take too long to go from 1 piece of equipment to another, the exercise won't be as effective.

Pros

■ The weather is not a problem.

■ You can adjust the equipment.

■ Machines provide feedback about your performance.

■ You can watch TV or listen to music or recorded books while you exercise.

Cons

■ You need access to a variety of machines.

■ You need to know how to use the machines properly in order to get a good workout.

Tips for circuit training:

■ Set up your program so that you alternate equipment that exercises your arms with equipment that exercises your legs.

■ For the best workout, do 4 minutes on each piece of equipment followed by 2 minutes of rest. On each machine, try to reach your target heart rate within 1-1/2 minutes and keep it there for the remaining 2-1/2 minutes.

DAILY TIPS AND ENERGIZING IDEAS

This section includes easy-to-do tasks, modifications to daily routine, and hints to enhance and reinforce the exercise in your aerobic regimen. Place little notes to yourself everywhere you tend to look during the day as reminders to do them from time to time.

AT HOME AND WORK

- Walk or bicycle to work or to shop. Walk to the subway, the train, or the bus. Get off public transportation several stops before yours and walk the remainder of the way. If you drive, park your car a distance from your destination and walk.

- Take the stairs instead of the elevator or get off the elevator several floors before yours and walk up the rest of the way. Do the same thing on your way down.

- If you normally exercise 15 minutes per day, gradually increase your exercise to 30 to 60 minutes per day.

- If you can afford to buy your preferred piece of exercise equipment, you can exercise more regularly because you won't need to go to a health club or watch the weather. Since you have the equipment at home, you can exercise while you watch TV. Other family members can also use the equipment.

- Do chores such as raking leaves briskly, to make them more aerobic.

- If you normally sit in your office 8 hours a day, get up every 45 minutes and power walk down the hallway for 5 minutes or climb several flights of stairs. You can even power walk to and from the break room and restroom.

- If you normally get up from your chair 6 or 8 times a day, get up 20 times instead and jog in place for 60 seconds.

- Jog in place during every commercial break while you watch TV.

- Walk energetically down the hall or down the street to speak to someone instead of using the phone or sending an e-mail.

- When you travel, stay at hotels with fitness centers or carry a jump rope in your suitcase, so that you can always get an aerobic workout.

GROOMING AND PREPARING MEALS

- While brushing your teeth, march in place as quickly as possible using a high-stepping gait.

- Jog in place for 30 seconds a few times while you prepare meals.

- While your food is cooking, power walk around the kitchen and living room or up and down the driveway several times.

- Jog in place for 60 seconds before and after you put on your socks and shoes each day.

(Get the idea? Every little bit helps!)

AT LEISURE

- Plan family outings and vacations that include aerobic activity, such as hiking, bicycling, or skiing.

- Walk the golf course instead of using a cart.

- Play singles tennis; it is more aerobically demanding than doubles. If you play doubles, you can increase your endurance (as well as your competitive readiness) by jogging lightly in place while you wait for play to continue.

- Include aerobic games such as racquetball and paddle tennis in your exercise regimen.

- Build time for swimming laps into leisure time at the pool.

- Don't just chaperone your child's skating or swimming party— take part in the activity.

- Enroll in a dancing or spinning class.

Weight Loss, Body Fat, Exercise, and Life Expectancy

Obesity can shorten your life. A study in the *Annals of Internal Medicine* found that being overweight and obese was associated with significant decreases in life expectancy. The loss in years is as follows:

- Overweight 40-year-old female nonsmokers lost 3.3 years.
- Overweight 40-year-old male nonsmokers lost 3.1 years.
- Obese 40-year-old female nonsmokers lost 7.1 years.
- Obese 40-year-old male nonsmokers lost 6.7 years.
- Obese female smokers lost 13.3 years.
- Obese male smokers lost 13.7 years.

To determine whether you are overweight or obese, you can calculate your Body Mass Index (BMI) using the following formula:

$$\left(\frac{\text{weight in pounds}}{\text{height in inches}^2} \right) 703$$

- BMI below 18.5 = underweight
- BMI of 18.5 to 24.9 = normal weight
- BMI of 25 to 29.9 = overweight
- BMI of 30 and above = obese

Can exercise help? Many studies cite the beneficial effect of exercise for weight reduction. A study in the *Journal of the American Medical Association* reports that regular exercise, such as brisk walking, resulted in reduced weight and body fat in a group of overweight and obese postmenopausal women. The walking program was of moderate intensity and done for at least 45 minutes, 5 days a week for 12 months.

A study in *The Annals of Internal Medicine* found that attempted weight loss was associated with lower mortality.

Exercise Type and Intensity

An article in the *Journal of the American Medical Association* looked at the relationship of intensity of exercise to actual risk reduction. Running, weight training, and walking were each associated with reduced risk of CHD. The study included the following statistics:

■ Men who ran for 1 or more hours per week had a 42 percent risk reduction of CHD.

■ Men who trained with weights 30 minutes or more per week had a 23 percent risk reduction.

■ Men who rowed 1 hour or more per week had an 18 percent risk reduction.

■ Men who walked briskly 30 minutes or more per day had an 18 percent risk reduction.

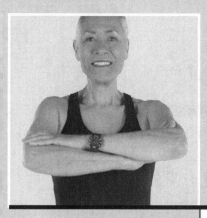

Chapter 7

Putting It All Together

Tricking Yourself Into Fitness: Exercising On Days When Your Body Resists

Some days you're lucky if you get 15 minutes to yourself. When you don't have time for a complete workout or you're tempted to skip a day, try these tricks:

- Do a wall slide while you brush your teeth.
- If you live in an apartment building, walk 2 flights of stairs and then take the elevator the rest of the way.
- Use a speakerphone or headset when you talk on the phone, so that you can do arm or leg weight exercises at the same time.
- Hold a plank/push-up position for 1 minute.
- Set your watch and walk for 7 minutes, then turn around and walk back to your starting point in 7 minutes. Once you reach the 7-minute mark, you should try to extend your time.

Can Exercise Help Depression And Mood?

Absolutely! A study compared exercise to medication for alleviating depression. The study found that a program of strengthening exercises, done 3 times a week for at least 6 weeks, was as effective as antidepressants.

Another study found that an 8-week strengthening program decreased anxiety and improved self-attentiveness and strength.

Another study looked at combining strengthening and aerobic exercise programs and felt exercise was a viable alternative to antidepressants for the treatment of depression; antidepressants may work more rapidly, but after 16 weeks, exercise was equally as effective.

Finally, a study looked at aerobic exercise alone and found that it decreased depression symptoms.

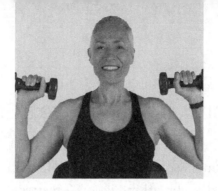

You must do the thing you think you cannot do.

—ELEANOR ROOSEVELT

Even positive lifestyle changes are challenging. But we see amazing people in our clinics every day, people of all ages and abilities, making astonishing strides toward fitness.

A COMMITMENT TO EXERCISE

Since making and keeping a lifelong commitment to an exercise program may be difficult, it is important to look at the factors that may affect your success. One significant factor is self-efficacy, the amount of self-confidence you have in your ability to perform an activity. To determine your self-efficacy, take this quiz. Use the following scale to define how certain you are that you will fulfill your exercise commitment:

I can exercise even when I am worried. _____
I can exercise even when I feel depressed. _____
I can exercise even when I feel tense. _____
I can exercise even when I am tired. _____
I can exercise even when I am busy. _____
Total score: _____

Very uncertain=1 point
Rather uncertain=2 points
Rather certain=3 points
Very certain=4 points

If you scored above 10, you are ready to commit to an exercise program. If you received a score of 10 or below, starting an exercise program will be more difficult, but *you can do it.*

ENCOURAGE YOURSELF TO EXERCISE

Starting and continuing a program requires effort. Take these hints seriously. Here are some ways to encourage yourself.

Breathe. Practice deep breathing if you feel stressed before you start exercising. Lie on your back with your feet on the floor, your knees bent, and your hands resting lightly on your lower abdomen. Take a deep breath in through your nose; feel your abdomen rise as air fills your lungs. Then exhale gently through pursed lips as the air leaves your abdomen. This technique will help you relax and focus.

Post reminders to yourself. Leave notes around your house to remind you to do certain exercises or to be aware of your posture.

Picture your goals. Choose a picture of someone you admire and would like to look like or a vacation spot you would love to visit. Put it in your wallet, on your office desk, or in a place where you will see it first thing in the morning. It will remind you why your exercises are so impor- tant. Copy exercises that are particularly important for you from this book and place them strategically around your home or office.

Be patient. Don't measure or weigh yourself too often; your body will not always change in a consistent, steady fashion.

Look in the mirror. Installing mirrors in strategic places—where you exercise, eat, dress, or bathe—may help you see the changes occurring in your body as a result of consistent exercise.

Reward yourself. Do something special for yourself as a reward for maintaining your exercise program. Rewards don't have to be expensive or fattening! Go to a movie with a friend. Allow yourself a Saturday of relax- ation rather than doing chores. Treat yourself to fresh flowers at the mar- ket. Take a long, relaxing bath. Choose a special article of clothing as an incentive to help you reach your goal.

Use visualization. Picture yourself succeeding and looking a certain way; it can facilitate your exercise performance. The more vivid the visualization, the better.

Use repetition. Develop a mantra in which you constantly repeat—out loud or in your head—the benefits of exercise ("improved posture, strength, balance, flexibility, and endurance") especially when you don't feel like exercising or if you feel like stopping once you've started. Positive reinforcement can put you back on the road to exercise. Keep telling yourself that you will look and feel better.

Make it social. Use exercise as a way to spend time with your friends and loved ones. Go for a walk together or take a bicycling vacation. Having company can be fun, reinforcing, and encouraging. If you make a commitment to exercise with someone else, you may feel a new sense of responsibility.

Have a schedule. As much as possible, exercise at the same time each day—usually the earlier the better. If you can't exercise early, head straight to the gym after work. If you miss a scheduled time, work it in at another time during the day or week.

Make it enjoyable. Listen to music or recorded books or watch TV while exercising. Or if much of your regular day is full of people and noise, take a quiet early morning walk.

COPING WITH SORENESS

Aches and pains due to exercise are normal. When you're stretching muscles or moving joints that you haven't worked in a long time, you should expect a degree of discomfort. Rest assured, you will feel better.

Typical treatments for such soreness include protection, rest, ice, compression, elevation of the affected body part, and, if necessary, an elastic wrap. You can soothe sore muscles using ice cubes and cold water in double-sealed plastic bags, a large bag of frozen peas wrapped in a thin towel, or commercially available reusable ice packs.

While some soreness is normal with the start of an exercise program, joint pain may be a cause for concern. If your joint pain begins to ease by the end of a week, it was probably a combination of muscle soreness and a sign that you may have overworked your body. As the soreness subsides, return to the offending exercise, but only at half the weight or repetitions. **Caution:** If you experience severe pain that lasts several days or a more moderate pain that lasts more than 2 weeks, contact a physician or physical therapist. If you experience any chest pain or shortness of breath when performing endurance exercises, consult your physician or cardiologist immediately.

PERSONAL EXERCISE EXPERIENCES

Art

Humorist Art Buchwald was unconscious for 10 weeks following a stroke in 2000. "When you awaken after that long, people expect you to look like Howard Hughes," he joked.

When Buchwald regained consciousness, he found the stroke had affected him both physically and mentally. He was referred to one of the authors for therapy. She tailored a program to his specific needs; it involved a warmup, stretches, strength training, gait training, balance exercises, tai chi, and proprioceptive training. He incorporated exercise into his life whenever he could. For example, he did a tai chi movement called "Crane Takes Flight" when he went through security at the airport, extending his arms outward and gently "flapping" them. Buchwald said, "People don't expect a person like me to talk about stroke. I'm a funny man, they think. But it's not all fun and games…. I use humor to face problems. I don't just write that way. I live that way." (Excerpts reprinted from *Your Health Magazine* with permission.)

Susan

When Susan, a music teacher, reached her fifth decade, she was as effervescent as ever but felt the years had taken their toll: she was worn out by the end of the day, had gained weight, and had developed diabetes. She had even begun to contemplate retirement. Her physician sent her to a physical therapist for education and an exercise program to slow or minimize the side effects of diabetes. Susan's goals were to continue teaching and to stop taking oral diabetes medication. She had never participated in formal exercise programs, though she walked and swam during the summer months. Working with her physical therapist, Susan decided a walking program would be most beneficial and enjoyable for her. First she learned proper form, then she began walking 3 times a week for 20 minutes. Each week, she added 5 minutes to her total time until she was walking for 45 minutes. After she reached 45 minutes, she added a day each week to her schedule until she was consistently walking 6 days a week. She stretched for 8 minutes after each walk.

As Susan continued to exercise, she noticed she no longer suffered severe shortness of breath. Soon she began to lose weight, and her blood sugar improved.

Then she decided she was ready for the next step of her program—strength training. Susan started with a 1-repetition maximum for her major muscle groups, using elastic bands instead of weights. Her program initially took 45 minutes, but when she became comfortable with the bands and the routine, she could complete it in 20 minutes. She made a videotape of herself performing each exercise and used it as a guide; this made it easier to do the routine.

After 6 months, Susan had dropped 3 dress sizes; further improvement in her blood sugar levels meant she could discontinue her medication. Susan now has much more confidence and energy, exercises daily, and continues to teach.

Wendy

Wendy pursued her exercises with enthusiasm. She found some friends to walk with, and she stretches and strength trains while watching the news. After 2 months, all of her scores improved. After 3 months she got a perfect score on each test. Wendy now feels much more supple when driving and turning her head, and people compliment her almost weekly on her improved posture. She keeps up with (and sometimes surpasses) her teenage daughters in endurance and stamina.

James

James said he had fun determining his domain scores and designing his own program; however, the thought of actually doing the exercises was less pleasant. He took the self-efficacy test, scored below a 10, and realized that he needed to motivate himself. He wrote down the times of his favorite TV shows and only allowed himself to watch them if he was doing his balance, posture, strengthening, or endurance exercises. After a few weeks, he found certain TV programs worked better with certain types of exercises. He liked to do postural, balance, and stretching exercises while watching the morning and evening news; talk shows lent themselves beautifully to endurance. He found strengthening exercises were best done when he watched sitcoms.

This television approach helped James stick with his exercise routine. After 2 months, he started to feel the benefits of his exercises; he decided to evaluate his progress by re-testing himself. He had improved dramatically on many tests. After 4 months, he received near-perfect scores. He became more self-confident and organized a neighborhood walking program. He now feels better about both his physical and social well-being.

WHAT ABOUT YOU? — CONTACT US

How is your plan working? Let us know how you do. We'd love hearing what works and what doesn't, about your successes and your trials. You can share your stories with us at authors@agedefyingfitness.com.

REFERENCES

CHAPTER 1

Barnes, D. E., et al. 2003. A longitudinal study of cardiorespiratory fitness and cognitive function in healthy older adults. *Journal of the American Geriatrics Society* 51(4): 459-465.

Beissner, K. L., et al. 2000. Muscle force and range of motion as predictors of function in older adults. *Physical Therapy* 80(10): 556-563.

The Cooper Institute, *Physical Fitness Assessments and Norms,* 2000, pages 84-86 and pages 92-94.

Cooper, K. H. 1968. A means of assessing maximal oxygen intake. Correlation between field and treadmill testing. *Journal of the American Medical Association* 203(3): 201-204

Csuka, M. and D. J. McCarty. 1985. Simple method for measurement of lower extremity strength. *American Journal of Medicine* 78(1): 77-81.

Di Bari, M., et al. 2004. Thoracic kyphosis and ventilatory dysfunction in unselected older persons: an epidemiological study in Dicomano, Italy. *Journal of the American Geriatrics Society* 52(6): 909-915.

Fatouros, I. G., et al. 2002. The effects of strength training, cardiovascular training and their combination on flexibility of inactive older adults. *International Journal of Sports Medicine* 23(2): 112-119.

Foldarvi, M., et al. 2000. Association of muscle power with functional status in community-dwelling elderly women. *The Journal of Gerontology* 55(4): M192-M199.

Gaub, M.G., et al. Efficacy of balance and flexibility interventions in a frail female centenarian. *Journal of Geriatric Physical Therapy* 27: 1:04.

Martin, J. C., et al. 2000. Maximal power across the lifespan. *The Journal of Gerontology: Medical Sciences* 55(6): M311-M316.

Schonberg, M. A., et al. 2006. Receipt of exercise counseling by older women. *Journal of the American Geriatrics Society* 54(4): 619-626.

Thompson, L. V. 2002. Skeletal muscle adaptations with age, inactivity, and therapeutic exercise. *Journal of Orthopaedic and Sports Physical Therapy* 32(2): 44-57.

CHAPTER 2

Bassey, E. J. 2001. Exercise for prevention of osteoporotic fracture. *Age and Ageing* 30-S4: 29-31.

Cutler, W. B., et al. 1993. Prevalence of kyphosis in a healthy sample of pre- and postmenopausal women. *American Journal of Physical Medicine and Rehabilitation* 72(4): 219-225.

Eagan, M. S., and D. A. Sedlock. 2001. Kyphosis in active and sedentary postmenopausal women. *Medicine and Science in Sports and Exercise* 33(5): 688-695.

Fritz, J. M., et al. 1997. A nonsurgical treatment approach for patients with lumbar spinal stenosis. *Physical Therapy* 77(9): 962-973.

Gregg, E. W., et al. 1998. Physical activity and osteoporotic fracture risk in older women. Study of osteoporotic fractures research group. *Annals of Internal Medicine* 129(2): 81-88.

Heinonen, A., et al. 1996. Randomized controlled trial of the effect of high-impact exercise on selected risk factors for osteoporotic fractures. *Lancet* 348(9038): 1343-1347.

Hertel, K. L. and M. G. Trahiotis. 2001. Exercise in the prevention and treatment of osteoporosis: the role of physical therapy and nursing. *The Nursing Clinics of North America* 36(3): 441-453.

Kado, D. M., et al. 2004. Hyperkyphotic posture predicts mortality in older community-dwelling men and women: A prospective study. *Journal of the American Geriatrics Society* 52(10): 1662-1667.

Kado, D.M., et al. 2005. Hyperkyphotic posture and poor physical functional ability in older community-dwelling men and women: the Rancho Bernardo study. *The Journal of Gerontology: Biological sciences and medical sciences* 60(5): 633-637.

Kelley, G. A., et al. 2002. Exercise and lumbar spine bone mineral density in postmenopausal women: a meta-analysis of individual patient data. *The Journal of Gerontology* 57(9): M599-M604.

Kudlacek, S., et al. 1997. The impact of a senior dancing program on spinal and peripheral bone mass. *American Journal of Physical Medicine and Rehabilitation* 76: 477-481.

Nelson, M. E., et al. 1994. Effects of high-intensity strength training on multiple risk factors for osteoporosis fractures. A randomized controlled trial. *Journal of the American Medical Association* 272(24): 1909-1914.

Nowakowski, P., et al. 1996. Lumbar spinal stenosis. *Physical Therapy* 76(2): 187-190.

Siddiqui, N. A., et al. 1999. Osteoporosis in older men: discovering when and how to treat it. *Geriatrics* 54(9): 20-32.

Sinaki, M., et al. 1996. Can strong back extensors prevent vertebral fractures in women with osteoporosis? *Mayo Clinic Proceedings* 71: 951-956.

CHAPTER 3

Adams, K. J., et al. 2001. Progressive strength training in sedentary older African American women. *Medicine and Science in Sports and Exercise* 33(9): 1567-1576.

Bean, J. F., et al. 2002. The relationship between leg power and physical performance in mobility-limited older people. *Journal of the American Geriatrics Society* 50(3): 461-467.

Brandon, L., et al. 2000. Effects of lower extremity strength training on functional mobility in older adults. *Journal of Aging and Physical Activity* 8: 214-227.

de Jong, Z., et al. 2003. Is a long-term high-intensity exercise program effective and safe in patients with rheumatoid arthritis? Results of a randomized controlled trial. *Arthritis and Rheumatism* 48(9): 2393-2395.

Evans, W. J. 2000. Exercise strategies should be designed to increase muscle power. *The Journal of Gerontology: Medical Sciences* 55(6): M309-M310.

Fiatarone, M. A., et al. 1990. High-intensity strength training in nonagenarians. *Journal of the American Medical Association* 263(22): 3029-3034.

Fiatarone, M. A., et al. 1994. Exercise training and nutritional supplementation for physical frailty in very elderly people. *New England Journal of Medicine* 330(25): 1769-1775.

Fielding, R. A., et al. 2002. High-velocity resistance training increases skeletal muscle peak power in older women. *Journal of the American Geriatrics Society* 50(4): 655-662.

Hakkinen, K., et al. 2001. Selective muscle hypertrophy, changes in EMG and force, and serum hormones during strength training in older women. *Journal of Applied Physiology* 91(2): 569-580.

Kelley, G. A. and K. S. Kelley. 2000. Progressive resistance exercise and resting blood pressure: a meta-analysis of randomized controlled trials. *Hypertension* 35(3): 838-43.

Melton, L. J., et al. 2000. Epidemiology of sarcopenia. *Journal of the American Geriatrics Society* 48(6): 625-630.

Ploutz-Snyder, L. L., et al. 2001. Resistance training reduces susceptibility to eccentric exercise-induced muscle dysfunction in older women. *The Journal of Gerontology: Series A, Biological Sciences and Medical Sciences* 56(9): B384-B390.

Saal, J. S. and E. Yurth. 1996. Nonoperative management of herniated cervical intervertebral disc with radiculopathy. *Spine* 21(16): 1877-1883.

Sullivan, D. H., et al. 2001. Progressive resistance muscle strength training of hospitalized frail elderly. *American Journal of Physical Medicine and Rehabilitation* 80(7): 503-509.

Wescott, W. L., et al. 2001. Effects of regular and slow speed resistance training on muscle strength. *Journal of Sports Medicine and Physical Fitness* 41(2): 154-158.

Williams, D. A., et al. 2004. Knee pain and radiographic osteoarthritis interact in the prediction of levels of self-reported disability. *Arthritis and Rheumatism* 51(4): 558-61.

CHAPTER 4

Arnold, C. M., et al 2005. The relationship of intrinsic fall risk factors to a recent history of falling in older women with osteoporosis. *Journal of Orthopaedic and Sports Physical Therapy* 35(7): 452-460.

Bell, A. J., et al. 2000. Characteristics and outcomes of older patients presenting to the emergency department after a fall: a retrospective analysis. *Medical Journal of Australia* 173(4): 179-82.

Bhala, R., et al. 1982. Ptophobia: phobic fear of falling and its clinical management: *Physical Therapy* 62(2): 187-190.

Burnfield, J. M., et al. 2000. The influence of lower extremity joint torque on gait characteristics in elderly men. *Archives of Physical Medicine and Rehabilitation* 81(9): 1153-1157.

Cheal, B. and L. Clemson. 2001. Older people enhancing self-efficacy in fall-risk situations. *Australian Occupational Therapy Journal* 48(2): 80-91.

Escalante, A., et al. 2001. Walking velocity in aged persons: its association with lower extremity joint range of motion. *Arthritis and Rheumatism* 45(3): 287-294.

Fansler, C. L., et al. 1985. Effects of mental practice on balance in elderly women. *Physical Therapy* 65(9): 1332-1338.

Furman, J. M. and S. L. Whitney. 2000. Central causes of dizziness. *Physical Therapy* 80(2): 179-187.

Gill-Body, K. M., et al. 2000. Relationship among balance impairments, functional performance, and disability in people with peripheral vestibular hypofunction. *Physical Therapy* 80(8): 748-758.

Hausdorff, J. M., et al. 2001. Gait variability and fall risk in community-living older adults: a 1-year prospective study. *Archives of Physical Medicine and Rehabilitation* 82(8): 1050-1056.

Hong, Y., et al. 2000. Balance control, flexibility, and cardiorespiratory fitness among older Tai Chi practitioners. *British Journal of Sports Medicine* 34(1): 29-34.

Legters, K. Fear of falling. 2002 *Physical Therapy* 82(3): 264-272.

Li, F., et al. 2005. Tai Chi and fall reductions in older adults: a randomized controlled trial. *Journal of Gerontology: Biological Sciences and Medical Sciences* 60(2) 187-194.

Mecagni, C., et al, 2000. Balance and ankle range of motion in community-dwelling women aged 64 to 87 years: a correlational study. *Physical Therapy* 80(10): 1004-1011.

Riemann, B. I., et al. 2003. Comparison of the ankle, knee, hip, and trunk, corrective action shown during single-leg stance on firm foam and multiaxial surfaces. *Archives of Physical Medicine and Rehabilitation* 84(1): 90-95.

Sattin, R. W., et al. 2005. Reduction in fear of falling through intense tai chi exercise training in older transitionally frail adults. *Journal of the American Geriatrics Society* 53(7): 1168-1178.

Skelton, D.A. 2001. Effects of physical activity on postural stability. *Age and Ageing* 30: S4: 33-39.

Tinetti, M. E. 2003. Clinical practice. Preventing falls in elderly persons. *New England Journal of Medicine* 348(1): 42-49.

Wolf, S. L., et al. Reducing frailty and falls in older persons: an investigation of Tai Chi and computerized balance training. 1996. *Journal of the American Geriatrics Society* 44(5): 489-497.

Wolf, S.L., et al. 1997. The effect of Tai Chi Quan and computerized balance training on postural stability in older subjects. *Physical Therapy* 77(4): 371-381.

Wu, G., et al. 2002. Improvement of isokinetic knee extensor strength and reduction of postural sway in the elderly from long-term Tai Chi exercise *Archives of Physical Medicine and Rehabilitation* 83(1): 1364-1369.

CHAPTER 5

American Geriatrics Society Panel on Exercise and Osteoarthritis. 2001. Exercise prescription for older adults with osteoarthritis pain: consensus practice recommendations. A supplement to the AGS Clinical Practice Guidelines on the management of chronic pain in older adults. *Journal of the American Geriatrics Society* 49(6): 808-823.

Bandy, W. D., et al. 1997. The effect of time and frequency of static stretching on flexibility of the hamstring muscle. *Physical Therapy* 74(10): 1090-1096.

De Deyne, P. G. 2001. Application of passive stretch and its implications for muscle fibers. *Physical Therapy* 81(2): 819-827.

Feland, J. B., et al. 2001. The effect of duration of stretching of the hamstring muscle group for increasing range of motion in people aged 65 years or older. *Physical Therapy* 81(5): 1100-1117.

Ottawa Panel. 2004. Ottawa Panel evidence-based clinical practice guidelines for electrotherapy and thermotherapy interventions in the management of rheumatoid arthritis in adults. *Physical Therapy* 84(11): 1016-1043.

Ottawa Panel. 2005. Ottawa Panel evidence-based clinical practice guidelines for therapeutic exercises and manual therapy in the management of osteoarthritis. *Physical Therapy* 85(9): 907-971.

Overend, T. J., et al. 2000. Cardiovascular stress associated with concentric and eccentric isokinetic exercise in young and older adults. *The Journal of Gerontology: Biological Sciences and Medical Sciences* 55(4): B177-B182.

Penninx, B. W., et al. 2001. Physical exercise and the prevention of disability in activities of daily living in older persons with osteoarthritis. *Archives of Internal Medicine* 161(19): 2309-2316.

Shrier, I. 1999. Stretching before exercise does not reduce the risk of local muscle injury: a critical review of the clinical and basic science literature. *Clinical Journal of Sport Medicine* 9(4): 221-227.

Westby, M. D. 2001. A health professional's guide to exercise prescription for people with arthritis: a review of aerobic fitness activities. *Arthritis and Rheumatism* 45(6): 501-511.

CHAPTER 6
American College of Sports Medicine. 2000. *Guidelines for Exercise Testing and Prescription 6th ed.* Baltimore: Lippincott Williams & Wilkins.

Dolgener, F. A., et al. 1994. Validation of the Rockport Fitness Walking Test in college males and females. *Research Quarterly for Exercise and Sport* 65(2): 152-8.

Gregg, E. W., et al. 2003. Intentional weight loss and death in overweight and obese U.S. adults 35 years of age and older. *Annals of Internal Medicine* 138(5): 383-389.

Heyward, V. H. 1998. Advanced Fitness Assessment and Exercise Prescription 3rd ed. Champaign, IL: Human Kinetics.

Irwin, M. L., et al. 2003. Effect of exercise on total and intra-abdominal body fat in postmenopausal women: a randomized controlled trial. *Journal of the American Medical Association* 289(3): 323-330.

Kasch, F. W., et al. 1966. A comparison of maximal oxygen uptake by treadmill and step-test procedures. *Journal of Applied Physiology* 21(4): 1387-1388.

Noonan, V. and E. Dean. 2000. Submaximal exercise testing: clinical application and interpretation. *Physical Therapy* 80(8): 782-807.

Peeters, A., et al. 2003. Obesity in adulthood and its consequences for life expectancy: a life-table analysis. *Annals of Internal Medicine* 138(1): 24-32.

Tanasescu, M., et al. 2002. Exercise type and intensity in relation to coronary heart disease in men. *Journal of the American Medical Association* 288(16): 1994-2000.

Wilk, B. R. and M. M. Valdez. 2004. When should physical therapists inform their patients their running shoes have run out—before it's too late. *Orthopedic Practice* 15:1:03.

CHAPTER 7
Blumenthal, J. A., et al. 1999. Effects of exercise training on older patients with major depression. *Archives of Internal Medicine* 159(19): 2349-2356.

Callahan, C. M., et al. 2005. Treatment of depression improves physical functioning in older adults. *Journal of the American Geriatrics Society* 53(3): 367-373.

Coyle, C. P. and M. C. Santiago. 1995. Aerobic exercise training depression symptomatology in adults with physical disabilities. *Archives of Physical Medicine and Rehabilitation* 76(7): 647-652.

Mather, A. S., et al. 2002. Effects of exercise on depressive symptoms in older adults with poorly responsive depressive disorder. *British Journal of Psychiatry* 180: 411-415.

Meland, E., et al. 1999. The importance of self-efficacy in cardiovascular risk factor change. *Scandinavian Journal of Public Health* 27(1): 11-17.

Perrig-Chiello, P., et al. 1998. The effects of resistance training on well-being and memory in elderly volunteers. *Age and Ageing* 27(4): 469-475.

Singh, N. A., et al. 1997. A randomized controlled trial of progressive resistive training in depressed elders. *The Journal of Gerontology: Biological Sciences and Medical Sciences* 52(1): M27-M35.

Stewart, K.J. 2002. Exercise training and the cardiovascular consequences of type 2 diabetes and hypertension: plausible mechanisms for improving cardiovascular health. *Journal of the American Medical Association* 288(13): 1622-1631

PERMISSIONS

Figure 2.1, page 26
Reprinted from *Mosby's Medical, Nursing and Allied Health Dictionary,* 5th edition, Figure A2. Kenneth N. Anderson, Revising Editor; Lois E. Anderson, Consulting Editor and Writer; Walter D. Glanze, Consulting and Pronunciation Editor. © 1998 Reprinted with permission from Elsevier.

Figure 2.2, page 26
Reprinted from *Musculoskeletal Examination,* page 431. Written by Jeffrey Gross, MD; Joseph Fetto, MD; and Elaine Rosen, MS, PT, OCS. © 1996 Reprinted with permission from Blackwell Publishers

Chart 1, page 28
Bone Measurement Institute, Merck & Co., 1996

Figure 2.3a and 2.3b, page 29
Reprinted from *Scoliosis: Diagnosis and Management,* page 25. Written by Rene Cailliet. Reprinted with permission from F. A. Davis Company.

Figure 3.1, page 67
Reprinted from *Mosby's Medical, Nursing and Allied Health Dictionary,* 5th edition, Figure A9. Kenneth N. Anderson, Revising Editor; Lois E. Anderson, Consulting Editor and Writer; Walter D. Glanze, Consulting and Pronunciation Editor. © 1998 Reprinted with permission from Elsevier.

Figure 3.2, page 68
Reprinted from *Mosby's Medical, Nursing and Allied Health Dictionary,* 5th edition, Figure A8. Kenneth N. Anderson, Revising Editor; Lois E. Anderson, Consulting Editor and Writer; Walter D. Glanze, Consulting and Pronunciation Editor. © 1998 Reprinted with permission from Elsevier.

Figure 4.1, page 155
Reprinted from *Mosby's Medical, Nursing and Allied Health Dictionary,* 5th edition, Figure A24. Kenneth N. Anderson, Revising Editor; Lois E. Anderson, Consulting Editor and Writer; Walter D. Glanze, Consulting and Pronunciation Editor. © 1998 Reprinted with permission from Elsevier.

Figure 5.1, page 190
Reprinted from *An Illustrated Atlas of the Skeletal Muscles,* 2nd edition, page 30. Written by Bradley S. Bowden and Joan M. Bowden © 2005. Reprinted with permission from Morton Publishing Company, Denver, CO, www.morton-pub.com.

Figure 6.1, page 232
Reprinted from *Mosby's Medical, Nursing and Allied Health Dictionary,* 5th edition, Figure A5. Kenneth N. Anderson, Revising Editor; Lois E. Anderson, Consulting Editor and Writer; Walter D. Glanze, Consulting and Pronunciation Editor. © 1998 Reprinted with permission from Elsevier.

Figure 6.2, page 232
Reprinted from *Pathophysiology of Heart Disease: A Collaborative Project of Medical Students and Faculty*, 3rd edition, page 58. Edited by Leonard S. Lilly, MD. ©2003. Reprinted with permission from Lippincott, Williams & Wilkins.

Figure 6.3, page 233
Reprinted from *Principles and Practice of Cardiopulmonary Physical Therapy*, 3rd edition, page 46. Edited by Donna Frownfelter, MA, PT, CCS, RRT and Elizabeth Dean, PhD, PT. © 1996 Reprinted with permission from Elsevier.

Figure 6.4, page 234
Reprinted with permission from EnchantedLearning.com

Indexes

• • ■ ■ ■

INDEX

ABOUT THE MODELS

DOMINIQUE A. NERO is a 22-year veteran instructor in the fitness industry, starting her career in 1983 as a part-time aerobics instructor. After retiring from a full-time corporate position in 1999, she has become certified in personal training, yoga, Pilates, water aerobics, and senior fitness.

In 1983, **SHEILA PAYNE**'s physician advised her to avoid strenuous physical activity because of degenerative discs in her back. After researching her options, she became a certified water aerobics instructor and began walking 3 to 4 miles a day. She then joined a local running club and has since completed several half marathons, both 5k and 10k runs, and a triathlon. She teaches stretch and flex, tai chi, yoga, and water aerobics to the elderly, and recently won gold medal and silver medals in the Atlanta Senior Olympics.

After a lower back injury in 1982, **ROY ALEXANDER** established a regimented exercise routine to strengthen the muscles around the injured disks and prevent the need for an operation to repair the damage. He has successfully avoided the operation by working out every day, his routine consisting of aerobic exercises, stretching, and weight training.

AUTHOR ACKNOWLEDGMENTS

The authors are greatly indebted to Lorne Jaffe for his invaluable assistance in early manuscript editing; his English and communication backgrounds enabled us to translate our normally clinical writing styles into language more easily accessible to our audience.

It has been a pleasure for both of us working with the staff at Peachtree Publishers, and we are indebted to them for their good judgment, their insightful and discerning reviews, and their continued encouragement throughout this process.

We owe special thanks to Margaret Quinlin, who was the first one we approached with the idea of doing this book and who stayed with us throughout its evolution with unwavering support.

We are especially grateful to Kathy Landwehr, whose editorial skill transformed our writings into this final published book.

We would also like to thank Linda Schaeffer and Kelly Mills for their photography; Marian Gordin, Phyllis Mueller, Vicky Holifield, and Elizabeth Snow for their editorial work; and Melanie McMahon Ives, Loraine Joyner, and Robin Sherman for their assistance with production and design.

And finally, thanks to Linda Schaeffer for locating the three wonderful AGE-DEFYING FITNESS models.

ABOUT THE AUTHORS

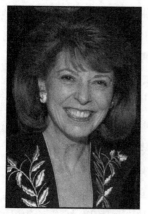 **MARILYN MOFFAT** has been in private practice for forty years and currently practices in the New York area.

She holds degrees from Queens College and New York University and is a professor of physical therapy at New York University.

Dr. Moffat has served as editor of *Physical Therapy,* the official publication of the American Physical Therapy Association.

She served as the president of the American Physical Therapy Association for six years, as well as a member of the APTA board of directors and as president of the New York Physical Therapy Association. Dr. Moffat is currently a member of the board of trustees of the Foundation for Physical Therapy and of the executive committee of the World Confederation for Physical Therapy, as well as an Associate of the Council of Public Representatives of the National Institutes of Health.

Dr. Moffat is a Catherine Worthingham Fellow of the APTA. In 2004, she was named the Mary McMillan Lecturer, the American Physical Therapy Association's highest award. She has been the recipient of many other awards, including the APTA's Marilyn Moffat Leadership Award, the APTA's Lucy Blair Service Award, the WCPT's Mildred Elson Award for International Leadership, the Ambassador Award from the National Strength and Conditioning Association, and the Howard A. Rusk Humanitarian Award from the World Rehabilitation Fund. The New York Physical Therapy Association named its leadership award after her.

She has given over 800 professional presentations, and she has taught and consulted in Taiwan, Thailand, Burma, Vietnam, Panama, and Hong Kong.

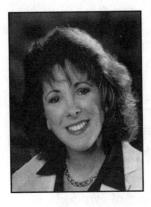

CAROLE B. LEWIS has been in private practice in Washington, D.C. since 1981. She has worked in home health, long-term care, acute hospitals, rehabilitation departments, and outpatient clinics.

Dr. Lewis holds master's degrees in public administration and gerontology from the University of Southern California and a PhD in health education from the University of Maryland. She currently serves on the medical faculty at George Washington University as a full adjunct professor in the department of geriatrics.

Dr. Lewis has published extensively in the field of aging. Her articles have appeared in *The Journal of the American Physical Therapy Association, Clinical Management, Geriatrics, Geritopics,* and *Senior Patient.* She is also the editor of the journal *Topics in Geriatric Rehabilitation.* In addition to her articles and journals, Dr. Lewis has written numerous textbooks on aging.

She is a Fellow of the American Physical Therapy Association. Dr. Lewis has received the APTA's Lucy Blair Service Award, the Clinical Excellence Award, and the Joan Mills Award, the highest honor from the Section on Geriatrics. She has served as the president of both the D.C. chapter and the Section on Geriatrics of the American Physical Therapy Association.

Dr. Lewis has lectured extensively, speaking in more than 46 states as well as in Israel, Australia, New Zealand, Japan, Finland, Canada, and China.

This book should contain a postcard that can be mailed to Peachtree Publishers to receive your free Thera-band. (The postcard is bound into the book after this page.) If you purchased this book and the postcard is missing, please call our customer service department at 1-800-241-0113, or e-mail *customerservice@peachtree-online.com* and use "Thera-band Request in lieu of Postcard" as your subject line. Please keep your receipt to confirm your purchase of a new book.

Thera-bands are also available for purchase from a number of online and brick-and-mortar retailers. For your convenience, we will keep a list of sources for the bands at our website for this book: *www.agedefyingfitness.com*.

We hope you enjoy the book and find it helpful. Here's to your good health!

Peachtree Publishers
1700 Chattahoochee Avenue
Atlanta, GA 30318
customerservice@peachtree-online.com
1-800-241-0113